Injured Mind,

Shattered Dreams

Brian's Journey From Severe Head Injury to a New Dream

D1413105

Janet Miller Rife

Library of Congress Cataloging–in–Publication Data

Rife, Janet Miller.
Injured Mind, Shattered Dreams: Brian's Journey From Severe Head Injury to a New Dream/ Janet Miller
Rife
p. cm
Includes bibliographical references and index.
ISBN 0-914797-95-6
1. Rife, Brian. 2. Brain Damage— Patients—United States.
–Biography. I. Title
RC387.5.R54R54 1993
362.1'968'0092—dc20
[B]   93-43284
                                                                                      CIP

10 9 8 7 6 5 4 3 2 1

Book and Cover design by Maria Teresa Guevara.
Cover made with lettering drawn from one of Brian's first letters during his recovery from the accident.

If you want to order this book call or send a letter to:
BROOKLINE BOOKS
P.O. Box 1046, Cambridge, MA, Tel (617) 868-0360 Fax (617) 868-1772

To Brian

To Sharon,
Share our journey!
Janet Miller Rife

Royalties from the sale of *Injured Mind, Shattered Dreams* will be applied to the long-term supported housing arrangement that meets Brian's and his family's needs.

Table of Contents

•

Chapter 8
EPILOGUE
157

•

•

• • •

Author's Acknowledgments

I am grateful to the many people who said to me, "You should write a book." One of the first was Neil Henry, the talented <u>Washington Post</u> reporter who wrote our story as a four-part series in June 1986. After the <u>Post</u> story, which included excerpts from my journal, I heard the same words from many friends, neighbors, and professionals who had worked with Brian. Among those voices were the women of my book discussion group. We'd begun to meet in 1984, reading and discussing many books from then till 1987. Those lively discussions and studies of authors' lives helped to break down the "author mystique" for me, a high school graduate with less than a hundred recent college credits. I doubt that I could have envisioned myself writing a book without the background of the "Ladies of the Club." (We had named ourselves after this best-selling novel of the mid-80's.)

Thanks to my husband Curt, who has grown emotionally throughout this journey and generously helped with housework during the writing. He lived graciously with the oddity of a wife who goes to bed at 8:00 p.m. in order to get up at 4:00 a.m. to write, helped me untangle the technicalities of word-processing, and encouraged me to persevere when my enthusiasm for the project lagged. Thanks to Brian's siblings Scott, Sheri, Eric, and Dan who have all made great strides in adjusting to the dramatic changes in our family and have helped me to maintain balance during these last eight years.

Brian has always been thrilled that a book was being written about him. Reading the early versions of the manuscript was one of the ways he began to learn what happened to him. His courageous spirit, his will to live, his desire to be all he can be and to give back to his community, all have inspired me to believe in the importance of telling the story. In addition Brian has made many helpful suggestions on manuscript content and on the book's title.

A special thanks to the two women whom I have seen as spiritual directors at different stages of the journey, Rhoda Nary of the Shalem Institute for Spiritual Formation and Sister Marian Hahn of the Cenacle. Both unfailingly encouraged me to believe in the work as a legitimate exercise of a God-given gift, during times when discouragement or questioning set in. I am grateful to the faithful friends in my spiritual support group, Pat Gauthier, Dottie Rossi, Diane Jenc, Loyes Spayd and Rosalie Shipe, who have shared their joys, sorrows, prayers and laughter with me over these many years. Diane and Dottie helped with the decision on the final wording of the title of this book. Rosalie, who was with me at the very beginning at the Dominican Retreat House, and at Shock-Trauma in Baltimore, has shared this journey in a most personal way.

I also wanto to thank Isolde Chapin of Washington Independent Writers, who encouraged me in the early stages of the book and later when I needed assistance with editing and shaping the raw material of my journal and tape recordings. With her help, I found Mary De Nys, an English professor at George Mason University. Mary's intuitive insight into my book, combined with her professional language skills, made her contribution especially significant.

Thanks also to Milton Budoff, my publisher, and his son Nathan, who encouraged me to reflect again on the emotions I experienced during early stages of our story. Milton's suggestion to have more input from Brian resulted in the interviews that form Chapter 7. A very special thanks to Theresa Rankin for her sensitive questions that helped Brian to express his version of events recorded in this book.

From the first day I decided to write a book in August 1986, I've sought places of quiet retreat to write, pray and reflect. My thanks to those who have provided such space in the last seven years. In Washington, I have appreciated the Madonna House and the Shalem Institute for Spiritual Formation; in Virginia, the Dominican Retreat House and the Cenacle; in Maryland, the Dayspring Retreat Center.

Thanks also to Maria Guevara of Brookline Books, who typeset the manuscript and patiently added last minute changes and additions. Thanks to my son Eric, manager of a photo shop, for his advice about processing the photos included in the book.

It is impossible to list all the people who have touched our lives in the years since Brian's injury. They are family members, persons with brain injury, and many professionals. All of these people are part of the book; without this collective experience, the story could not have been told.

• • •

Foreword

Injured Mind, Shattered Dreams is an account of a journey, a journey about the lives, roles and relationships of a family that experiences one of life's most feared events, a tragic accident that leaves a loved one permanently disabled. This is a story about love, about the struggle to survive, about a family coming to terms with loss, and finally about a mother's effort to get the "system" to respond to her son's changing needs.

Along the way there are constant mini events or crises which cause the Rife family and Brian to adjust their expectations for recovery and to come to understand the lack of a "solution" to the problem of brain injury.

Injured Mind, Shattered Dreams is must reading for neuro-psychologists, rehabilitation specialists, caregivers, and anyone interested in human drama. I found the book compelling and moving.

The events surrounding a head injury are instant and demanding. One instant you are a normal person with your dreams and hopes for the future, the next instant you are fighting to survive and then comes the long journey of recovery, rehabilitation, and the adjustments that must be made to new expectations.

For many parents and loved ones, experiencing this loss results in chronic sorrow, a grieving that never goes away. In Injured Mind, Shattered Dreams, Janet and the Rifes share their grieving and their joy. This is a parent's perspective, especially a mother's viewpoint. In the process, the family discovers there is no final solution. There are just new "sets of challenges." But what makes this book so compelling is the way in which the Rife family and Brian come to terms with each new challenge. The ultimate victory is learning to cope, learning that interdependence is something all of us experience and need in order to live satisfying lives. As the book ends the reader comes to realize there is no ending, just new beginnings.

As the President of the National Head Injury Foundation, which is dedicated to improving the quality of life for persons with head injury and their families and to promoting prevention of head injury, I believe Injured Mind, Shattered Dreams will be very helpful as a resource for the more than two millions Americans who sustain a head injury every year.

By George A. Zitnay, Ph.D
President , National Head Injury Foundation , Washington D.C.

. . .

Preface

I am struck with how silently true success comes. Often we expect victory to have a public nature. The local football team, the politician who wins the election, the athlete from the home town who excels is typically published in the local newspaper with numbers, scores and record breaking identifiers included. But every day I see those who have had a head injury achieve victory. There are no crowds, no scores, and the newspapers don't even notice. Yet they achieve victory just the same. Even the injured person may not recognize the victory because his/her expectations are focused on a different target. I have come to call the injured person's success a "silent victory." Each and every day in hospitals, treatment programs, job settings, and homes, people with head injury and their families navigate silent victories; victories that must have inherent value and victories that must apply to their lives and times; victories that underscore how they have come to apply themselves in their world and in their time.

For many years now, going back to the 1970's we have been able to help people survive catastrophic head injuries. In fact, we professionals even measured our success by how many people survived. In the intervening years we have come to learn that although our ability to help people survive has improved, our ability to help them live fully again requires ongoing attention. I have seen many injured individuals and their families look at the "ones in the know" with bewilderment and disbelief. However, I have also witnessed, in spite of our technological lag, individuals who not only survive but learn how to live again. Every day I have seen people who are injured not only improve their skills, but learn to apply themselves anew. In fact I have come to redefine success in neurorehabilitation, and recovery from brain injury, by how well the persons can apply themselves in their world. Application of skills and the application of oneself in self care, self protection, home life, productive activities and social settings now stands as the operational definition of success.

How the injured person and his/her family experience this journey through silent victories has not been adequately captured. We have studied family reactions, individual needs and use of professional services, but we have not captured the experiential curve of recovery. The victory of self application relies on a great many influences well beyond the early phases of skill re-development. Many non-traditional caretakers have contributed to such silent victories. Most of all those who have achieved a level of victory have some insight into what has made them a success in others' eyes. If we could capture these insights from those affected, the families and the injured person, we would find that some of the most valuable information on the subject may be in the minds and hearts of those this book describes.

In addition to the humane features of knowing "what others are going through," we professionals would be more precise in our application of treatment strategies, new medications and an array of helping techniques if we listened more closely to the injured person and to his/her family. Our need to collaborate in all we do would be enhanced and the victory of self application would be better served if we were able to coordinate the medical, social, and familial recovery curves by understanding the experiences of the injured person and the family helping to bring about those silent victories.

At the time of a head injury there is an explosion of events that drives us all in varied directions. Although we attempt to apply some order to the experiences by imposing levels and ideas of continuum on the process, sometimes we trick ourselves into believing that recovery is some neat linear progression that follows from one level to another. Although in the early phases of recovery, we can apply our helping efforts in some step-wise linear sequence, we cannot believe that learning to live again is so simplistic. The myth of linear progression towards victory at times confuses the injured person and his/her family when what they experience does not "match" our professional continuum. Services can be linear but recovery is multi-faceted and experienced as an array of questions and needs all simultaneously demanding solutions. When the injured person's experience coincides with what caregivers are doing we have improved collaboration and use of assistance, but when the experience of the individual varies radically from the assistance given, we have lost efficiency and created hurdles toward victory.

Psychology, philosophy, psychiatry, and religion are but a few of the approaches to studying the way we experience events. Gaining knowledge from the "experiencer," however, seems the heart of the issue. The seminal question, "Can we ever know?" may be unsolvable, but we cannot excuse ourselves from the responsibility of trying to know. The question of success in recovery and the ability to learn to apply oneself must be answered from the perspective of those taking the journey towards victory.

I have known the Rifes for many years of their journey. I have seen silent victories and I have seen disappointments. I have seen Brian come to understand the new "combination of traits" he calls Brian. I have seen a family system invest time, resources, and their very lives in helping Brian recover. I have known their questions about services. I recall most of all parents who adjusted their lives, roles and relationships to "help." I have seen bright, capable individuals struggle with helplessness. I have watched an individual, a family and a community try to make sense out of recovery from a traumatic brain injury.

This book captures the experiential side of the journey. From a mother's perspective, you will view a series of experiences, all revealing that recovery from a brain injury is not finite. Instead recovery is an unfolding set of problems to be solved. This family does not go from having a problem to being problem free. Instead, as Brian improves he now qualifies for a new set of problems, disguised as opportunities. The mixed blessing of improvements places Brian and his family in a new arena of events and outside of their previous "comfort zone." Getting well means qualifying for a new set of solutions and more discomfort. As environments change, new skills need application and the constant interface between skill application and new environments constitutes recovery and ultimately victory. Much like raising a child, the parents and family learn that each new developmental phase poses new problems and requires new solutions.

In some ways the term "solution" is inaccurate. The real problem of living with a brain injury is better defined as coping, coping with both opportunity and lack of opportunity. The solution to emancipation issues for Brian, his siblings and parents is a two-way street–all are being emancipated at all times with the ultimate solution being an *interdependence that works*. As the reader will note, aside from the technical points of recovery and the academic knowledge learned during the Rifes' journey, the persistent need to solve the interdependence issue permeates each page. At times they use knowledge, at times they hold onto beliefs and values and they always try to find a way to hold onto each other. Not letting anything or anyone "slip through the cracks" becomes a major task. The effort to save others while holding onto oneself becomes an over-riding effort during this journey.

It is important to realize that this journey does not differ significantly from the journey many have navigated. The Rifes' growing knowledge, skills, excitements and disappointments parallel thousands of individuals and their families' efforts to succeed. The difference is in the ability to communicate the experience in a manner that helps the reader understand. Although the experience in <u>Injured Mind, Shattered Dreams</u> is an individual one, take this journey with the Rife family in order to learn about your own journey and the experience of many.

Again, do not confuse the book's ending with a solution or an end to the journey. Victories, however many, do not leave everyone feeling good. There remain many more solutions to be reached, more opportunities to endure, and more time together to be navigated. What you take away with you is not solutions; instead you take away ideas about how Brian and his family coped, adapted and endured opportunity and disappointment. Most of all you gain some working knowledge of the experience for Brian and his family and a new understanding of the existential nature of recovery and the interdependency necessary for "silent victories." As the book ends, the reader will realize that many experiences will be left unpublished, that one can live with brain injury and that life does continue.

by Peter Patrick, Ph.D
Director Learning Services, Shanandoah Campus

· · ·

Author's Introduction

I grew up in Loretto, a small western Pennsylvania town, molded by the images and values of the Roman Catholic church. Jesus dying on the cross, suffering and tortured, was present in the prayers and rituals of my childhood. Regularly I recited the words of the creed at Mass in the Romanesque St. Michael's Church, built in 1899, "He was crucified under Pontius Pilate; he suffered, died and was buried. On the third day he rose again..." High above the altar, another image dominated, a living, radiant Jesus, surrounded by angels escorting him through the clouds as his followers looked up in awe. This central mythology of my religious experience enabled me to expect a resurrection when Brian was near death, both for him, and for us, in the midst of our suffering. For Brian, would that mean a resurrection in the afterlife or a resurrection in this earthly life? Some of the prayers and readings that sustained me during the most difficult times reflect this central question.

As a child, I learned of saints like Father Damien, who followed Christ's example of compassion for people cast out from society. Damien left a world of comfort to live on Molokai, a remote island in the Hawaiian chain, to become one with lepers, abandoned because of their diseased bodies. Because Damien and others like him were among my childhood hero images, perhaps it was easier to transcend my fears of being with people who at first seemed different and to gradually accept that Brian would indeed be different in his new life.

During the sixties and seventies, I developed a passion for social justice by studying the lives of spiritual and national leaders like Dorothy Day and Martin Luther King, Jr. Catholic social teaching, sometimes referred to as "our best kept secret," declares: "Every human is a person, endowed with intelligence and free will, who has universal and inviolable rights and duties." (John XXIII) This core principle informed my conviction that a terrible injustice was occurring when Brian's life was saved through modern technology, but no system was in place to provide for the quality of that life. As a mother who felt a sense of participation with the Creator at the birth of each of my five children, I felt compelled to fight for Brian's life with all my strength, in spite of the fact that his negligent behavior led to his brain injury.

I would not claim that all my actions in the last eight years have been motivated by lofty spiritual motives. Sometimes, I've been willful, judgmental, and controlling. "Put away your sword, Janet," I remember saying to myself once when I realized I was still being combative while a different attitude was called for. The intuitive reader will no doubt see these aspects in my perspective of events.

On July 13, 1985, the day before this story begins, during a conference at the Dominican Retreat House, the retreat director, Father Calvin, discussed the Chinese word for crisis: a combination of two symbols, one meaning danger and one meaning opportunity. After July 14, we were in danger of losing Brian, of losing faith, of being destroyed financially and emotionally. As we continued to walk this journey, we began to see the opportunities to inform others about the silent epidemic of head injury, to impact on the delivery of services, to stress the need for prevention, to grow in understanding and solidarity with other persons with disabilities and their families in our communities.

Within days of Brian's injury, I began keeping a journal because I was terrified by what was happening to us and believed that writing down my feelings, perceptions, and prayers as they came to me would be therapeutic. As we felt overwhelmed by conferences with doctors and specialists at the shock-trauma unit at the University of Maryland Hospital, we asked permission to tape these meetings. These tapes and my journal were the raw materials that enabled me to write this book.

Months later, when financial, rehabilitation and ethical issues occupied our minds relentlessly, we began to realize the magnitude of the brain injury epidemic and became aware that our experience was only one of thousands. Brian's story is typical of many survivors of traumatic brain injury, but each survivor will have a different experience. As the mind of each person is unique, so too the injured mind.

During the months of struggle with Kaiser-Permanente to obtain funding for Brian's rehabilitation, Kaiser was often perceived in my mind as an "enemy." In retrospect, Kaiser personnel were merely a reflection of a larger issue, the many doctors and other health care professionals who are uninformed about this new group of survivors and the quality of life that is possible for them with appropriate treatment. Twenty years ago, Brian could not have survived his injury. In the 90's, intense debate rages about how rehabilitation after brain injury should be delivered. Articles in the New York Times in March and April of 1992 examine fraudulent practices in the rehabilitation industry and highlight newer models that shorten in-patient treatment.

It is my hope that our story will dissolve some of the fear and mystery surrounding brain injury and leave readers with a new respect for the vulnerable, but incredibly resilient brain, still the least understood part of the human body. Further I hope this story can be used by those who are engaged in research to create the best, most cost-effective ways to rehabilitate persons with brain injury and other diseases that affect the central nervous system. Counselors, clergy and caring friends who want to learn how to best assist the family of a person with brain injury may also find our story instructive.

Brian, who wanted to be a pilot, has become a pilot of a different sort, finding a path through dark and confusing territory, holding tenaciously to life, and ultimately displaying courage, perseverance and a sense of humor that have captivated many professionals, friends and audiences along the way.

August 1993

Note: In Injured Mind, Shattered Dreams, I frequently use the word "survivor" for people who have survived a traumatic brain injury. As a writer, I generally subscribe to the "person-first" language guideline, which would indicate "person with brain injury" as a better choice. However, another guideline is that people with a particular disability have the final say about words used to describe them. As of this writing, most people with brain injury whom I've met prefer the term "survivor," and have named their voice of leadership within the National Head Injury Foundation (NHIF) the National Survivors' Council.

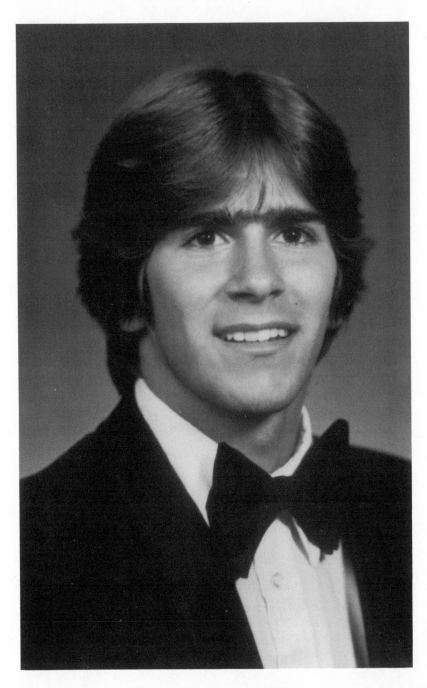

Brian's graduation, June 1985

.1.

SHOCK-TRAUMA

The Dominican Retreat House,
McLean, Virginia

Saturday, July 13, 1985

A bright flame burns from the oversized candle in the middle of the altar, the light of Christ, surrounded by small unlit votive candles. Blue, yellow, red–all the shades and variations of our humanity, seeking to be rekindled by the One who is the Light. The reader speaks soothingly the words of the Twenty-third Psalm:

> *The Lord is my shepherd, I shall not want;*
> *In green pastures he gives me repose;*
> *Beside still waters he leads me;*
> *He refreshes my soul.*
> *Even though I walk in the valley of the shadow of death,*
> *I will fear no evil.*
> *For you are at my side, with your rod and your staff*
> *that give me courage.*

One by one, the retreatants enter the reconciliation room[1] to sit facing the priest, to receive the grace of this ancient sacrament, to be reconciled to our God, creator, redeemer and spirit. As each woman returns to the chapel, she lights a small candle from the flame of the larger one. Gradually a multicolor glow emerges, a spirit of peace settling on the group. The retreat director invites us to meditate on the 23rd Psalm as we walk silently to our rooms.

• • •

---

1. In a reconciliation room, the penitent and priest usually sit face to face in contrast to the pre-Vatican II Confessional.

The decision to take part in this retreat was made rather suddenly. Two friends had been planning it for some time, but I had remained indecisive. As the date came closer, circumstances seemed to direct me to go. My husband, Curt, and our two youngest sons, Eric, 13, and Danny, 9, had driven to Florida for a ten-day vacation with grandparents. Brian, 20, home from college for the summer working construction and Sheri, 18, would be home alone. My '78 Omni with its MS RIFE license plates sat in the driveway. Brian drove it to his summer job, and we'd set no particular guidelines about its use at other times. I taped the phone number of the retreat house to the microwave and left, free of anxiety about how the two of them would spend the weekend.

Sunday morning, July 14

After morning prayer and a nourishing breakfast of pancakes, fruit and coffee, we gather in the conference room for a brief social period before the first talk of the morning. Petite white-robed Sister Amy, with her smile of inner joy, leans through the doorway and says, "There's a phone call for Janet Rife." I pick up the phone in the small office near the entrance. It's my daughter Sheri. "Brian has been in a car accident –near Salisbury, Maryland– he and Tom were on their way to Ocean City –a helicopter is taking him to Baltimore– they said he is in critical condition." Then, between sobs, "Don't worry, he'll be OK." She gives me a number to call at Peninsula General Hospital where Brian was first taken by ambulance. I tell her I'll be home as soon as possible and hang up.

In seconds sympathetic voices surround me. I make a weak protest to Rosalie and Joan, the friends I'd come with, "You don't need to give up the rest of your weekend." But in minutes, I melt into complete dependence on the actions of others. Suitcases packed, goodbyes spoken, we leave the shelter of the retreat house to face a vast unknown. They think and decide for me on the way to Springfield. We won't try to contact Curt, now somewhere between Florida and Virginia. We'll ask Ken, a neighbor, to meet Curt at the house. Eric and Danny can stay overnight with friends. Rosalie and her husband will call for directions to the University of Maryland Hospital and lead the way, while my 22-year-old son Scott and I follow in his car.

When we arrive in Springfield, I find myself functioning on my own again. We reach Scott by phone in Manassas. While we wait for him, we piece events together with Sheri. "Some of the guys were here last night; David and his girl friend and Tom Kilday, they drank a few

12-packs of beer. I went to bed about midnight. Brian came down to my room later and said he and Kilday were going to Ocean City. About 8 o'clock this morning I got a phone call and I couldn't figure out what to do. I didn't see the phone number of the retreat house at first. I called David and he said I'd better get in touch with you as soon as possible. Then I saw the number."

We learn that Tom survived the crash with only a few bruises; his parents picked him up from Peninsula General Hospital a few hours after his arrival.

"Just Tuesday," Scott says, as we head on to Route 95 for the 75 minute drive to Baltimore, "we were out in the carport, working on the motorcycle. We were really in touch with each other; best talk we've had in a long time."

I reflect back on a scene in the kitchen July 3, the day after Brian came back from Virginia Tech orientation. He had met some of the AFROTC staff and been measured for his cadet uniform. "Y'know," he said to me, as he leaned against the counter in the kitchen, "just yesterday there were colonels and majors shaking my hand—I was somebody—today I'm back picking up trash on the construction site!" He shook his head at the irony and turned to search the refrigerator for an afternoon snack.

Scott, entering his fourth year at Virginia Tech, had been looking forward to showing Brian around Blacksburg when he transferred to Tech in September. As we move along the highway in his Subaru, we do not speak of what is happening inside us; we're trying to stay calm. Underneath my heart, a box forms, its lid tightly sealed, holding in the demon emotions that would pull me into chaos.

Panic pushes violently at the closed lid of this box when we are out of the car on our way in to the imposing structure on Greene Street in inner-city Baltimore, the University of Maryland Hospital. We ask directions to the shock-trauma unit and wind our way to the lowest level of the aging building. We've already heard that this shock-trauma unit is considered one of the best in the country, and we hold that idea firmly as we pass halls of empty boxes, scarred walls, a boiler room and finally enter the shabby family waiting room, with its aging divans and stained carpet in about 12 square feet of space. I mechanically fill out some forms while the clerk addresses us, "The trauma team will be down to talk with you in a few minutes."

The spokesman for the trauma team is Dr. Schlegel, a neurosurgeon with a boyish demeanor. His words, though gently spoken, describe harsh reality.

"Brian has suffered severe brain trauma.There is an instrument inserted in his skull that measures cranial pressure. A tracheotomy tube has been inserted in his throat allowing him to breathe with the aid of the respirator.We will begin surgical procedures on him soon that will last about three hours.We'll just have to wait and see. He is in a coma, and at this point the prognosis is poor. You can go up to see him now."

The high metal bed sits in a hallway waiting for a space in the Critical Care Recovery Unit (CCRU). Approaching with tentative steps, I see a "Frankenstein" version of my son –the left side of his head is shaved and something called a "subarachnoid screw" is sticking out of his skull.It is covered with surgical tape and protrudes about four inches.The hair remaining on his head is stiff, mannequin-like, from dried blood. A trickle of blood and other material (brain matter?) cascades from his right ear. His arms are rigid by his side. A pencil-sized tube has been inserted at the base of his neck. His chest moves in a steady rhythmic movement, the respirator breathing for him. His face is relatively intact, only a few stitches on his chin and above his right eyebrow. I touch the beautiful eyebrows, dark and full; yes, it is Brian. The nurse says it's OK to kiss him. I do, as if in a dream. Then we leave him and return to the waiting room. Scott and I hold on to each other as anguish rushes out of the box. One of us says, "How could he be so dumb, why didn't he take care of himself!"

I find the meditation room and try to pray. Here in this tranquil surrounding, another box forms alongside the box of demons beneath my heart. I ask for courage, acceptance, hope, whatever gift God can plant in this new box to neutralize the frightful energies in the other. I picture Brian in the hospital bed, consider the artificial look of his body, and wonder if his spirit has already left him, moving down the path to the next life. Will he come back to tell us of this experience or go on? Who is there to meet him? I think of Gangya, Curt's grandmother who died nine years ago at the age of 90. My spirit finds some comfort in these images.

Back in the waiting room, Curt and Sheri have arrived with Ken Bounds. Later, Curt would recall his reactions to Ken's shattering news. "I first thought he was joking, but then I looked at his eyes and I knew this was no joke. I guess I had to be the macho man, so I said, 'Let me clean up and change clothes first.' I then did the practical thing, called the auto and health insurance companies to tell them what I knew, which was not much."

Soon after Curt's arrival, Dr. Schlegel reappears to tell him personally about the seriousness of Brian's condition. Curt asks, "If he lives, if he pulls through this, what are we talking about, a vegetable?" Schlegel said yes, but immediately added that Brian could surprise everybody. We are asked then, with apologies for the seeming insensitivity, if we would be willing to donate Brian's organs for transplant. We are stoic, "Yes, that would make sense."

Another member of the trauma team comes into the waiting room and informs us:

> "We will not be able to perform the three-hour surgery at this time. When Brian's head hit the windshield, his brain crashed against the inside of his skull. As a result of that trauma, his brain is now swollen. If we tried the surgery, his head would literally explode. The oral surgeon will stabilize his loose segments; then we'll wait for the swelling to subside. In the meantime, the supply of oxygen to his brain is being cut off. Brain cells die under such circumstances and do not replace themselves."

Terror and confusion rage inside the box; I fixate on the odd words used to describe my son –*explode, loose segments.*

Brian has no injuries to his internal organs or broken bones in other parts of his body, but his head took tremendous impact: a shattered jaw, broken bones in his face, and fractures on the front and left side of his head, one of which extended to the base of his skull.

Around 12:30 that night we see him again briefly, now in the CCRU, a formidable room of computer terminals, tubes and wires. At the center of the room is a nursing station surrounded by twelve beds. We avert our eyes from the others and follow directions to Bed 11, where we touch Brian. Only the feel of his warm flesh reassures; all else invites chaos. If the lid of the box flings open now, I will become a mad woman, screaming at the fates, tearing out my womb. "She is holding up very well," intone the voices that taught me how women behave when confronted with the cruel episodes of life.

After one o'clock we fall exhausted into the beds prepared for us at Curt's brother's house in Columbia. Curt and I grip each other tightly as waves of grief wash over us, the deadly reality of the day's events all-consuming. The images of the 23rd Psalm quiet the demons in the box. As the Frankenstein image of Brian crashes in to my consciousness, my mind insists "green pastures and still waters." Somehow I sleep.

My youngest son and I sit on the living room couch. We have been advised by family services to be honest with Brian's brothers and sisters about his condition and let each decide freely about visiting him. Slender, brown-eyed, sensitive Danny asks, "Is Brian going to die?" I say, "It is very serious and he may die, but they will do all they can for him." Danny, so much like his brother Brian ten short years ago, decides stoically to see his brother. I explain how he will look –the pressure screw in his skull, the stitches, the trach tube –achieving a matter–of–fact tone that makes me feel like a recorded message.

Sheri, only 18 months younger than Brian, knows quickly that she wants to see him. Eric decides he prefers not to go. He has a close friend whose only brother died after an auto crash that obliterated the lower half of his face. She preferred to remember her brother as he was before the accident. We honor Eric's decision.

Tuesday, July 16

We arrive at the fourth floor, Sheri, Danny, Scott, Curt and I, and line up outside the CCRU to outfit ourselves in the necessary gowns and caps. We joke a bit about how great we look, and it breaks the tension. Visits are limited to 10 minutes, and as we leave, we are asked to sit down with a staff member. She explains that we can make a tape of family voices for him, "Sometimes things are getting through even when there is no visible response." We answer a few easy questions: what were his hobbies, his work, his favorite music, was he in college? Then, "How does he react to crisis?" We look at one another and search for the answer. The times when a family argument was taking shape, the times when a friend had hurt him or treated him unfairly ran through our thoughts. The only obvious answer, "He tends to withdraw." We gradually absorb the awareness that this didn't feel like a "good answer;" to come through something like this, one had to be a "fighter."

When we leave, I decide we should all go to the chapel and make a tape for Brian. The strain begins to break in. Scott thinks I'm trying to run the show. I think they're copping out on Brian. We reach an uneasy truce. On the trip home, a lively conversation develops when the tape recorder is turned on, good spontaneous family talks.

> "Remember in Belgium when we went down to the Chateau D'Havre and threw rocks in the moat. You threw a big one and fell down the hill with it and cut your head!"

The tape is filled with reminiscences of adventures from our 1970-73 stay in Europe and laughter, worthy to be taken to Brian on our next visit.

In my bed that night, as I remember the cuts, scratches, bruises, the near misses of Brian's 20 years, the pain has me again in its grip, not unlike the contractions of labor, surging, rolling and gradually subsiding.

I can't stop touching my other children; I need to feel the smooth, healthy skin of their arms, see the life in their eyes, experience their wholeness, see them moving freely.

Wednesday, July 17

I am straightening the house; Curt's parents are coming from Florida. Two friends have come to help, their intuitive antennae up for my emotional needs. In the downstairs bathroom, my eyes rivet on the waste basket still piled high with empty beer bottles. Rage comes rushing up to my throat; I long to smash these accomplices to our pain, one by one, to hear the delicious sound of their destruction. Robot–like, I carry them in a paper bag upstairs and present the evidence to my friends, also the mothers of grown sons. They prod me, "Scream, shout, swear, let it out!" I stiffen and let loose an expletive hitting the air like a bursting balloon, a momentary release. The bottles lose their power as I walk quietly to place them in the outdoor trash receptacle.

That evening, Curt and his Mother and Dad go alone to the hospital. Eva Mae says when they return, "He squeezed my hand when I spoke with him!" But the nurse had cautioned, "It was probably only a reflexive movement," since they'd seen no other signs of conscious response.

Thursday, July 18

Several friends, all mothers, come to pray with me for Brian. In the morning I'd gone to Brian's bedroom for the first time since the accident and looked for items to make him more present to us as we pray. His red clay-stained denim cutoffs from his construction job, the folder from his recent orientation at Virginia Tech, his bow with its smooth dark wood and graceful curves (a present from us on his 17th birthday). And finally, leaping into my vision from the shelf, a hand-carved wooden fist Brian had created in a three-dimensional art class at Longwood College during the recent spring semester. I held it, turned it, felt its solidity, saw in its shape a symbol of hope, of will, saying "Fight, Brian."

All of these objects are placed on the round table in the center of our living room. We join hands and begin, "Our Father, who art in heaven, hallowed be thy name, thy kingdom come, thy will be done, on earth as it is in heaven..." Then we sit quietly, allowing images to come to each of us. I think of Brian as he had looked on the several occasions I'd seen him since the accident, of the chapel, of my wondering if he was on his way to the next life. Then something outside of my conscious thought process enters, a bolt of lightning seems to touch him and restore the life force, the energy to come back to us.

Another woman visualizes Brian in the hands of Jesus and Mary. A third focuses on the skill and dedication of the professionals surrounding Brian. A fourth, who had just heard the news, weeps, saying, "He has no idea what hit him."

In the afternoon my parents arrive from Pennsylvania, and Eric decides to see Brian. We don our gowns and hats, by now a familiar ritual, and enter the unit once again. My father grabs Brian's hand and says, "Brian," in a commanding tone, "squeeze my hand!" "He did it!" he says triumphantly. I remember the story of Eva Mae's experience the night before. Just a reflex, the nurse had said. "Probably just a reflex, Daddy," I say, feeling like a traitor. "I know the difference between a reflex and a squeeze," he says, his voice sure. I decide to try it. "Brian, squeeze my hand," I say in his ear. I feel the pressure on my hand. I am charged with electricity! After today's prayer session and the sensory overload of events, I do not trust my own judgment about what I feel or do not feel. But my father allows no doubt to enter his mind. Brian squeezed his hand. He tells the story again and again, his face glowing with pleasure. I remain "objective."

At home, my mind starts to race. If we are going to get Brian back, how much of him are we going to get back? They've said, "Many brain cells already dead and dying–they do not regenerate like other body cells." What does that mean? I remember exactly three terms from high school health class, the cerebrum, the cerebellum and the medulla oblongata. I begin crashing through the book shelf in the rec. room, encyclopedias, medical books, looking for some further explanation of what part of the brain does what, some bit of information to hang on to. I sleep with heightened anxiety, but in the second box beneath my heart, a tender seed of hope is planted.

The next day we receive a call that Brian is indeed responding to verbal commands, observed and recorded by various members of the CCRU staff. Scott, Danny, Curt and I go to see for ourselves; my parents have returned to Pennsylvania, "Grandpap" perfectly secure in the hand clasp he has experienced.

We are told the swelling has subsided and they have removed the subarachnoid screw. He is also now breathing one of three breaths on his own. "The life force *is* back in him!" I think as I look at him that night. His body lies in a more natural position, like the "real Brian" sprawled on his bed napping.

The nurse on duty that night, a solid woman with dangling pineapple–shaped earrings, speaks with us briefly. We touch Brian as though he is quite fragile and are unprepared when she yanks his leg roughly and demands, "Wiggle your toe for your Mom and Dad!" All eyes shift to the toe– it moves, unmistakeably. That night I dream of angels in pineapple earrings.

Saturday , July 20

At 7:30 this morning I run next door and tell our neighbors, "We're getting him back!" Their daughter Karen and her college roommate will visit Brian the next day.

Sunday, July 21

I've been given the name of Bill H. of the Virginia Head Injury Foundation. My words spill out in torrents to him on the phone, "Coma for five days, shock trauma, brain swelling, wiggled his toe." After he listens to me patiently for 20 minutes, I realize he's heard all of this a hundred times. He successfully plants two thoughts for me and Curt during the course of the conversation, "Take care of your own needs" and "remember you have other children." He also sows the seeds of understanding in me that this is indeed good news, but only the beginning of a long haul. His son, Bill says, has been in a coma for four years.

What does it mean to "take care of our own needs"–proper rest, food, normal conversations about things other than Brian? Bill tells me siblings come to the Head Injury Foundation meetings saying, "Not only did I lose my brother, I lost my parents too." I had thought of resigning my part-time job at Hogan & Hartson, a prominent Washington law firm. It seemed at first that I must devote myself fulltime to Brian's recovery, but after speaking with Bill, I decide against a sudden change.

I think about the coping mechanisms that have come to me. Oddly enough, since I am not a computer oriented person, the framework that presents itself in my mind is computer-like. *Input, output* and *function* describe aptly my method of getting through the days. Input–accept encouragement, help, sympathetic words from others. Output–give encouragement, understanding to others in my family and to friends of Brian who come to see us. Function–make my mind a blank and sweep the floor, do the laundry, buy milk and bread. This level, steady space between the boxes allows me to gather courage for the rollercoaster-like plunges and climbs ahead.

Monday, July 22

We visit shock-trauma in the evening, driven to Baltimore by a long-time friend, Monsignor Paul Lenz, who was the pastor in my home-town parish in the 50's. We talk with Brian, assuming that he hears and understands everything we say. Again Brian moves on command, his toe and his hand. We are elated, but this time other realities seem more evident. His arms are strapped to boards and punctured with intravenous lines; he is fed through a tube inserted through his mouth directly to his stomach. The tracheotomy tube protrudes from his neck and is covered with plastic tubing that connects with the respirator as well as oxygen and moisture. He is catheterized and urine empties into a bag at the side of the bed. The three of us pray with him before we leave. Msgr. Lenz treats us to dinner at the Inner Harbor; we allow ourselves to talk about other things.

Tuesday, July 23

Brian's high school buddy Jack Winstead visits. The night after the accident, Jack had driven impulsively to Baltimore at 3:00 a.m. to see Brian and had not been allowed into the CCRU without a family member. Jack's questions are direct, "There's a rumor that he is brain dead. Is that true?" "No, Jack, he is not brain dead– we don't know what damage his brain has sustained. There is no way to tell at this point."

Jack wants to know if it's OK for him to go to the beach. He decides to go if I promise to call if he's needed. He leaves his car for us to use, "The horn doesn't work, but if you push this little button here...and the left side door latch is stuck from the outside, but you can open it this way." Curt and I are warmed by his gesture and his youth.

Wednesday, July 24

I accept the offer of a ride to Baltimore from a friend. Today, Eric, Danny and I meet Brad Swanson, the speech pathologist who will be working with Brian. Tall, with intense brown eyes, a moustache, and a friendly smile, Brad becomes a significant person for Brian and for us during our stay at shock trauma. His job is to stimulate Brian to any kind of sensory or motor response, the most elementary being a consistent response to verbal commands: "Raise your forefinger; nod your head." A popsicle is his favorite prop. Cold and wet, it provides stimulation to Brian's lips. If he reacts, Brad can estimate what sensory information is getting through the brain stem to the higher functions. Brian is in a wheelchair when we arrive, his body stiff and robotlike, one eye open with a blank stare, the other closed, his mouth wired tight from the fracture.

Brad tests him for recognition. "Is this your Mom?" he asks. "Lift two fingers for *yes*." He did! "Are these your brothers?" Again, a *yes* response. Brad asks me to come nearer to the wheelchair, and he helps Brian to lift his left arm. He suggests I place myself under his arm. "Now give your Mom a hug," and I feel the pressure from his arm. The first of a long chain of bitter-sweet moments, pain and joy trying to mix like oil and water. Danny and Eric burst into tears and we leave soon after that. Brad suggests we bring in some family pictures for him to use during his sessions with Brian. The second box near my heart expands to receive another tender seed.

Thursday, July 25

Scott, Sheri, Curt and I arrive at the hospital for a conference with the team treating Brian. We wonder at our own brains' ability to process all this complex information, and we ask permission to tape the meeting. "The CAT scan taken yesterday shows only a moderate amount of swelling," we are told. The maxillo-facial surgeon says in a few days he will do "permanent fixation of the mandible [lower jaw]" if Brian's neurosurgical condition is stable.

The intern overseeing Brian's basic medical needs speaks next:

> "Brian's brain has taken a good bang and has to wake up. A simple-minded analogy –if you get punched in the arm, it gets black and blue. You don't do anything for it– you watch it. In that sense, we just have to wait and watch Brian's brain."

We are still looking for some information about what parts are damaged, what functions impaired. "What does the CAT scan show?" Curt asks,

> "It gives only anatomy, tells us about the presence or absence of swelling, clots, enlarging of the ventricles– doesn't tell anything about functional status. The best way to measure is what speech and physical therapy are doing." Brad adds, "The EEG shows how

brain waves are transmitted, lets us know if messages are getting
through the brain stem, which is like the on-off switch for access
to the higher brain functions."The potential for infection in fluid
cavities surrounding and within the brain and the facial sinuses is
a big concern. These cavities contain blood and fluid as a result
of the injuries Brian has sustained. The leakage of cerebrospinal
fluid concerned us, but that seems to have stopped. When fluid is
leaking out, it can also transport bacteria in. Brian is ready to be
moved to the intensive care unit (ICU) as soon as a bed is ready.
Overall, we're very satisfied with his progress. He has sustained
a very serious brain injury but appears stable."

Brad adds,

"Initially I saw only a very primitive response to light or sound, an
extending of the arm or leg in response to stimulus, which told us that
something was getting to the brain stem itself, but not beyond. Now
he is beginning to process more complex information. With a brain
injury like Brian's, you have to keep after him or he will just lie there.
Often response is best to familiar people, family and friends. Basically
I am really excited about his progress."

Dr. Schlegel, the diminutive neurosurgeon who spoke with us the
night Brian arrived in shock-trauma, speaks next,

"This qualifies in the near miraculous recovery stage already.
What we've seen has far outstripped what we ever expected. He
shows significant comprehension of what's going on around him.
How much better he's going to do, we still have no way of
knowing, but the progress so far is very encouraging indeed. It
will be a long road, and the degree of recovery is unknown to all
of us. It's unlikely he will stop here. He's made liars out of all of
us and I'm very happy."

Curt laughs lightheartedly and says as he shakes hands with Dr.
Schlegel,

"It was much nicer talking with you today."

I can hardly wait to get back to Springfield to tell all our praying
friends about Schlegel's "miracle" language.

Friday, July 26

Jack and another friend have returned from the beach and accompany Danny and me to Baltimore. We arrive to find Brian in the chair and Brad wielding the popsicle again. Brian's right eye is more fully open today, and the bluish bruise is beginning to fade. I say hello to him, then let Brian's friends move forward for a hand squeeze.

I'm aware of Brad's voice sounding like Mr. Rogers. "Do you want to hold the popsicle now? Put it up to your mouth. Come on, Brian." Then, "I'll bet you'd like to shove it up my nose!" Something approaching a smirk crosses Brian's face. We all laugh. It is a tremendously good sign— far more than the primitive response Brad had described earlier.

When I'm alone with him in the evening, thoughts of hope and miracles elude me as I rub his arms, his chest, his legs and wipe his face with a moist cotton pad. When I ask him if he remembers Jack and Jeff's visit that afternoon, he looks blank, unresponsive. He is to be moved to yet another room, so I decide to stay for the move, assuring that none of his things are left behind.

The man in the bed next to him in the new room brings to my mind medieval images of the souls suffering in hell. His small body is contorted grotesquely. A tube is stuck down his throat, his mouth wide open. He writhes from time to time. A black woman stands by his side, her face a mask. I ask if he is her husband. "He's my boy," she says, a faint smile crossing her face.

When the attendants lift Brian from the stretcher to his new bed, the muscles of my belly contract at the sight of him, saliva dripping from his mouth and fluid pouring from his nose, his body limp and seemingly lifeless. "Really exciting, very encouraging, miraculous," the experts are saying, but the words that make sense come from our friend Ken, speaking from the heart, "God damn, that's rough, seeing him like that— I know what you people are going through!"

Saturday, July 27

I awake this morning grieving. Surely the loving God of my understanding would not bring Brian so far and fail to bring him far enough for a meaningful life. I consider the awesome technology that snatches life away from death. Might death be more merciful? Easier to let go of him, to give him over to the next world rather than consign him and us to a half-life. But no, continuation of these thoughts I must reject. Then a comforting image comes to my mind. Brian is walking toward me, near perfect in his physique; he smiles and says, "Hi, Mom."

Wednesday, July 31

A meeting with the team is scheduled. Because we expect only more good news, we bring Danny along. We gather again in the small waiting room and hear a report from the maxillo-facial surgeon, "The jaw looks good–will be wired shut for six weeks."

Then we hear a long, rambling discussion from a nurse practitioner about rehabilitation. She deals with "time frames to be rehabilitated" and the range of possibilities from job training to nursing home, all couched in such ambiguous terms as to be nearly meaningless and utterly confusing.

The social worker describes her contact with a representative of Kaiser Permanente, our medical insurer, "Their coverage is great as long as Brian is here –they cover everything– but when he is ready for rehabilitation, they don't cover anything. So you need to check out some alternative sources of funding, vocational rehabilitation services or state aid in Virginia."

Dr. Greenberg, a neurosurgeon we'd not yet met, comes in, is introduced, sits down and begins explaining in ominous tones: "Before we can start thinking about rehabilitation, there is another major hurdle Brian has to get over." Curt and I sit, with Danny between us, gradually growing numb as he speaks. There is indeed a continuing leak of cerebral spinal fluid and it must be repaired. He speaks with slow, deliberate language.

> "It's a very risky procedure, the equivalent of three major operations. We will be exploring the entire lower half of his skull, working directly under the brain, near major blood vessels. We will explore the area to find the leak and repair it. It will take about eight hours and will probably be done tomorrow."

The lid closes harshly on the box where the seeds of hope were planted only a few days ago, denying light and oxygen to the tender shoots. We decide to call our parish priest in Springfield to come and administer the Sacrament of the Anointing of the Sick to Brian. I do not think of it as the "last rites," but rather a blessing and a prayer to carry us forward through whatever is to come.

We reach Father Curtis, ordained only a couple of years, idealistic, handsome, and young enough to still believe he can always respond to every need. I wonder, as we wait for him to arrive, if he has responded before to such a call in his brief experience. Soon we see him and Chuck McCoart, a candidate for the priesthood from our parish, walking toward us from the parking lot. Blonde Father Curtis and dark haired, moustached Chuck, glowing with wholeness and youth are a welcome sight.

Bits and pieces of information from conferences, visits, tumble out from Curt and me as we try to fill them in. "And this is the wooden hand he carved at school last year." "Yesterday he responded to yes/no questions." They look at us with the sympathy and pure feeling of the idealistic young, not yet seriously bruised by life's hard edges. They say we are an inspiration, "You're coping so well."

We go to the ICU where Brian is recouping strength after the facial surgery. Only one eye is visible and it is swollen shut. The rest of his face is bandaged and a surgical glove ice pack laying over his covered eye. Since there is a limit of four visitors allowed, Chuck waits outside. Curt, Danny and I go with Father Curtis to Brian's bedside for the sacrament. Father Curtis reads softly and tentatively:

> "We have come together in the name of our Lord Jesus Christ, who restored the sick to health, and who himself suffered so much for our sake. He is present among us as we recall the words of the apostle James: 'Is there anyone sick among you? Let him call for the elders of the Church, and let them pray over him and anoint him in the name of the Lord. The Lord will restore his health, and if he has committed any sins, they will be forgiven.' Let us entrust our injured brother Brian to the grace and power of Jesus Christ".

As Father Curtis anoints Brian with holy oil he prays, his voice gaining confidence, "May the Lord who frees you from sin save you and raise you up. Amen." Then we hold hands while touching Brian and pray as Jesus taught, "Our father, who art in heaven..."

Curt leaves the ICU so Chuck can come in. Chuck, four years older than Brian, knew him in school. Now he breezes in, confident in contrast to Fr. Curtis' uncertainty. He jokes with Brian, "Hey, you're looking good. I like the haircut, kind of a mohawk!" Then, without warning, Chuck keels over by the side of the bed, out cold. Father Curtis and I stare in disbelief. He grabs my arm, looks at his friend and says, "I don't even know what to do!" But the ICU staff does. They swoop Chuck up dispassionately and sit him in a wheel chair. As he comes to, his embarrassment hits. "I'm so sorry, I'm so embarrassed. We came to try to help out and this..." I put my arm around Chuck and say, "It's OK, all part of your training for the priesthood."

A jester has jumped into the space between the boxes, not exactly the angel of hope I'd imagined, but nevertheless a positive spirit. Whatever comes, death or recovery, we shall laugh again.

August 3

Three weeks have passed since Brian's injury. Because the neurosurgery had seemed extremely urgent, the next two days' delay is very frustrating. New and more critical cases are coming in to shock-trauma daily, and Brian's surgery is not considered urgent enough to be done ahead of these newly injured. We're invited to a small wedding, an old friend of Scott and Brian's, and we leap at the chance to do something "normal" and "happy." Never have I appreciated a wedding more. The bride smiles, her eyes are radiant. Life goes on.

Sunday, August 4

Curt and our neighbor Karen go to see Brian this afternoon. The bandages are off from the facial surgery, the stitches to be removed tomorrow. The surgeon comes in while Curt is there and says, "Post-op x-rays were positive." Curt reports that Brian was very active, moving all four limbs, "like he was trying to get out." He responded to some questions by nodding his head, memory in and out, regarding such questions as "Are you in the hospital?" No word yet on the neurosurgery. We are frustrated with the lines of communication and feel a little foolish at having panicked after the meeting with the team last Wednesday.

Monday, August 5

Two friends drive to Baltimore with me for a visit. Rosalie and I go in first, proceeding into the room holding hands only to find Brian's space empty. "Oh no, they've lost my kid," I say. We find him down the hall, at last in a more "normal" room, two beds and a TV. He is sitting up in bed. His right eye looks at me with real expression. It seems to twinkle; the blank empty stare is gone. I say, "Hi, Brian, you look great" and really mean it. Brad comes in shortly. I've come to love the sight of him, actually the only constant face over the last two weeks and the one who is most in touch with the essence of Brian, his spirit, his personality. Our hunger for the return of all of those parts is consuming.

Brad gives him a strawberry milkshake today. He squeezes a few drops into the corner of Brian's mouth and encourages him to suck in through his teeth and swallow. With a stethoscope he "feels" the swallow on the side of his neck. Brian accomplishes five or six swallows and we all applaud his efforts. Brad comments, "You have a regular cheering section!" Brian smiles. Brad gets out paper, clipboard, and pencil, asks Brian to write the number one and a two. He does a credible job; another chorus of approval. Then a black magic marker and some shapes, a square, a circle and a triangle. The triangle proves to be the hardest. Brad says soothingly, "That was pretty close." Brian is asked, "What month is it– October?" He shakes his head no. "May?" He shakes his head no. "June?" Again no. "August?" Brian nods yes. Another chorus of approval. What is the year? He shows 1 - 9 - 8 - 5 with his fingers, slowly but accurately. "All right!" intone the cheerleaders. More work follows with the letters of the alphabet, spelling "Rife" by identifying the correct letters and a little improvisation using hand signs. Brad says Brian is his star patient, and I realize an A in calculus pales in comparison to this compliment!

After Brad leaves, I ask Brian if we can say a prayer with him. He nods yes; I read a Navajo Indian prayer that seems to have been written just for us.

Prayer for Recovery of Mind and Body

Restore to me
my feet
my body
my mind
and my voice.
Take away your spell from me today,
remove your spell from me today.

You have taken it away from me!
It has departed far from me –
you have taken it far away from me.

I recover in a magnificent fashion.
My eyes regain their strength;
happily the spell is removed.
I walk without pain,
I walk with light within.
Thus happily you accomplish your works

In the chapel on the way out, we say a brief but heartfelt thank you. The seeds of hope are sending out new green shoots, nourished by the sunny warmth of this day.

Tuesday, August 6

Still no word on the neurosurgery. I work at Hogan & Hartson and have arranged to meet Msgr. Lenz and accept another ride to Baltimore after work. Brian is sitting in the chair when we arrive, his movements stiff and jerky. My overall feeling is more desolate than yesterday's warm images. I sit and talk with him for nearly an hour, amazing myself at the stream of consciousness that comes. When he leans forward, the fluid drips steadily from his nose. I find some pads in the cabinet and absorb it as I talk. "You remember Stacy; she got married on Saturday." He nods in understanding. Then I launch into the story of Stacy's sister Terry, backpacking in Colorado last week. Coincidentally she met some girls from Springfield and as they talked they discovered their common ground, proceeding to the "do you know..." stage. "Did you know Brian Rife?" the girls said, relating the story of his accident. Too much complexity for Brian to grasp; he looks quizzical. I move on to other chatter.

Wednesday, August 7

Finally, today the seven-hour craniotomy is completed. Curt and I both elect to go to work and wait till evening to receive word from Greenberg. The operation was successful, he reports, "We found the leak and were able to patch it with material from the undersurface of the scalp." Brian's skull had been opened from ear to ear with an S-shaped incision now held together by staples, the newest method of surgical closure.

Yet another new version of Brian. Now he is in a turban, covering the huge incision. I wonder how it looks and how it will heal. He is again unresponsive as his body recovers from this additional trauma, but we are prepared for and accepting of this temporary setback.

August 9-10

Allowing myself a few days respite in Pennsylvania with my parents, I suggest they make a tape for Brian after I explain recent developments. "Just a few words, anything you can think of."

Mother says,

"We're praying for you all the time, all our friends and the Franciscans and hope in a little while you'll be feeling better and come spend some time with us."

Daddy begins,

"Do you remember the time when you were just a little fella,

Grandpap took you into the bathroom and I thought you were high enough to stand and reach the commode. A little bit later I watched and here you went on the floor! You stepped back and you looked up at me and said, 'Oh no, not again!' And remember the time you went with me to Potter County, we did some fishing, and remember the deer and the coon, and that night the bear came in outside the camp. That was some excitement!"

Monday, August 12

Two friends of Brian's from Longwood have come to Springfield to meet us and visit Brian. Tall, lanky Mark Holland, with his southern drawl and down-home simplicity had been a special friend in the dorm. Mark had made the long drive from Charlottesville to Baltimore to see Brian the Sunday after the accident, bringing pictures of the gang from the dorm, taped to sheets of notebook paper and captioned in large letters. Mark's sense of what Brian needed was right on target. I learned later he had another brain-injured friend in his home town.

Today Mark and Jeff, another dorm friend, bring a poster they made for Brian. It's a picture of Vern, the bumpkin in the TV ads, and reads, "Hey Brian, Get Well Soon. Ya know what I mean!!!" The bandage is off Brian's head today. The incision travels from an inch above his right ear across the top of his head, then in a curve to just above the left ear, like the stitching on a baseball.

Mark's handling of the situation shows maturity beyond his years. Jeff is hard-pressed to hide his shock at seeing his once carefree, handsome friend in such a state. We get almost no response from Brian, no indication that he is aware of our presence in spite of persistent talking, urging, and cold washcloths applied to his forehead.

Thursday, August 15

During a meeting with the team, Dr. Greenberg expresses his satisfaction at the success of the craniotomy and makes some hopeful statements, "Obviously, no contact sports or roughhousing for at least a year or two until the skull fuses again. The bone has to knit together, but swimming, walking, jogging– all that is OK."

However, Brad Swanson and social worker Bernice Wolfson are more cautious, "It's impossible to predict how much the accident has impaired Brian's mental abilities. Unlike stroke damage, which is usually limited to one portion of the brain, a closed head injury like Brian's can cause widespread damage." Brad says, "Brian is going to look very normal from the outside in another week, once his hair grows back and his scars heal. But... we can't see the black and blue marks inside his head."

At the advice of the staff at shock-trauma, Curt and I visit a rehabilitation center near our home in northern Virginia, Mount Vernon Hospital in Alexandria. Mount Vernon is a modern facility near George Washington's historic home. The characteristics of the building itself are a marked contrast to the shock-truma unit in Baltimore. We are relieved when we walk inside. The spacious lobby is decorated with dozens of peace lilies, their dark green, broad leaves shining and conveying a feeling of growth and warmth; clear, wide hallways and everywhere windows–air, light and space softening the blow as we encounter people in wheelchairs with spaced out expressions, withered limbs, others staring at plates of food. But even that first day, staff members make an impression –happy, upbeat people who like what they are doing, I think. The equipment for people with disabilities is impressive, and we comment appropriately but struggle with acceptance of the notion that this is a place for Brian, who only one month ago had been a strikingly handsome, healthy young man.

August 17-18

Space to recoup our energies, examine what's going on at home in Springfield, get Eric and Danny registered for their fall soccer seasons. I meet with Rose F., the mother of a young woman who has made a good recovery from a severe brain injury. Her daughter had wrecked her car when she was seventeen, suffering internal injuries, a broken pelvis, a crushed left arm, in addition to a closed head injury. She tells me of the long odyssey of Donna's recovery. How she searched all over the country to find an adequate head injury rehabilitation facility for her daughter. How she dropped everything and went to Boston with Donna. when she was accepted at Lewis Bay, spending fifteen hours a day working with her daughter, refusing to accept any negative prognoses.

> "They told me she would never walk again, that her IQ would never go above 50. I read everything I could about the brain, I learned every connection, every nerve ending, and made it my business to know exactly what was going on at all times. If any drug was being administered to Donna, I looked it up in my own copy of the <u>Physician's Desk Reference</u> and made sure I understood any possible side effects."

After her daughter left Lewis Bay in Massachusetts, she spent a whole year in therapy in Virginia.

"I drove her every day to therapists in the area and worked with her myself. I wouldn't let anyone near her who didn't have a positive attitude."

Rose goes on to explain other challenges,

"There is often a combative stage that people recovering from a head injury go through; even proper older women may let out a string of obscenities. But this is actually a good sign, because it means that some of the emotional function is returning. There is also often a loss of inhibition; someone admired Donna's blouse so she took it off and offered it to her! It is very much like growing up all over again, a telescoping of the process that takes place from birth to adolescence: learning to eat, to use the bathroom, to be socially appropriate."

My mind is barely able to process this new but vital information, but I tuck it away for later reference.

Rose also suggests a practical measure to be taken for Brian immediately, "Does he have any high-top sneakers? Get them on him right away, right there in the hospital bed. They help prevent foot drop. It's a weakening of the muscles in the foot that occurs when a person is bedridden for a long time." She gives me some printed information about the Head Injury Foundation and some articles on brain injury.

A few days later we have a chance to meet her daughter. We marvel at her wholeness and learn that she has been able to resume her job with Hechinger's and will re-enter college soon.

Tuesday, August 20

Neighbor Ken Bounds drives my parents to Baltimore today. Curt and I have an appointment to visit the Woodrow Wilson Rehabilitation Center (WWRC) in Fishersville, VA. We look over the brochures as we head south on Route 95 and encounter another new batch of terminology, physiatrists[2], neuropsychologists, rehabilitation engineers, adaptive equipment specialists, work adjustment programs. The complexity of recovery from a brain injury begins to sink in.

---

2. Physician who specializes in physical medicine and rehabilitation.

We meet briefly with a staff member and are told where we can wait for the next tour given by a volunteer. We resolve to speak to every disabled person we meet, an effort to grasp the realities of Brian's condition and what his future needs might be. Confronting our prejudices and misunderstandings, we must begin the process towards acceptance.

We are less shocked this time when we encounter wheelchairs, computers that allow a person with impaired vision to read complex material by magnifying it on a screen, specially equipped cars that provide a simulated driving experience. After we've finished the tour, we walk alone, holding hands, across the grassy quadrangle surrounded by dormitories for the higher functioning patients at WWRC.

We see ahead of us a young man walking. He takes two or three steps that appear normal, then his equilibrium deserts him and he staggers from side to side, forward and back, like the proverbial drunken sailor. Then his balance takes hold once again, and he proceeds with normal steps. Transfixed, we watch this process repeat itself several times. When we reach him, I say hello and we introduce ourselves. He is Mike and he speaks to us appropriately. We tell him we are heading back to the main offices where we are to meet with someone in admissions and we've gotten a little turned around –can he direct us. He says, "Sure, I'm going that way right now. I hope you'll be able to keep up with me, I am in a hurry."

Curt and I look at each other, feeling as though we've entered the twilight zone again, and respond, "Sure, we'll be able to keep up with you, Mike. Thanks for your help."

As we walk, Mike tells us a bit about himself.

> "I just got back to Woodrow last month. I was here before, but I was violent. I got a lot of beatings when I was a little kid and sometimes I would just be violent with the therapists and nurses. So I had to leave for a while. Now I'm back again and this time I'm going to make it."

When we arrive at the door of the Admissions Office, Mike waves goodbye and continues on his arduous way. The realization that Mike had probably suffered his brain injury at the hands of his own parents makes us grateful for the lives we have.

We meet briefly with the admissions counselor and are told there is a year waiting list for brain injury survivors. They can tell us very little about possible financing if Brian is accepted at Woodrow Wilson. We are given several phone numbers if we wish to be back in touch at the next stage in Brian's recovery.

We finish dinner (brought in by neighbors) that evening with my parents, who've been to see Brian in the afternoon. Just after dessert, Mother takes a deep breath and says she has some bad news. "The nurse told us today that Brian is going to need another operation... there's another leak of the fluid," she says, barely holding back the tears. "We didn't want to tell you right away. You needed a little time to relax first." Having had no official word of this, we are disappointed that my parents were told in such an off-hand way. We all assume this means opening up Brian's skull once again.

The box under my heart, once strong in containing its "demons," is cracking and breaking now from the strain. It releases a flow of grief as Curt and I lie together in bed. We don't name the emotion or speak of our mutual gratitude for the release, but the moment strengthens us.

Wednesday, August 21

A meeting has been arranged with the team at shock-trauma. Dr. Greenberg explains,

> "He is still leaking spinal fluid, from the one spot we could not reach with the previous surgery, right in front of the brain stem. I've just talked with the otolaryngologist [ear/nose/throat surgeon] and we can go in through the sinuses, through the nose into the center of Brian's head. We will patch the area where the fracture is."

Reviewing the films from the most recent CAT scan, he continues,

> "We will do it tomorrow, should take about four hours. None of these operations are short. This should not set him back too much, but it means another week before he can be transferred to Fairfax Hospital. There are always some risks with a general anesthesia, but we think they are minimal. Always a risk of infection with an operation, but the risk is a lot less than not doing the operation."

We are relieved that it does not mean opening Brian's skull again. Greenberg goes on to explain:

> "Usually when we see a fracture in that part of the head, it means universal brain stem injury. He's the first that any of us can recall in a long time with this fracture who has survived. He probably does have some injury to the brain stem, but the CAT scan doesn't pick that up very well. There are about a hundred groups of

neurons connected to the brain stem, all microscopic; damage to any of them, even the size of a pin prick, might be enough to produce a significant problem. Ultimately we look to see how he functions. In about two more weeks, we'll be able to remove the wiring from his jaw."

Brad adds,

"Today it was really interesting. He was moving his lips a lot and he got really mad at me. I think if his mouth wasn't wired I would have gotten an earful. He's showing a lot of emotion, happiness, anger, frustration. His eyes are still dilated, not reacting to light."

Curt asks, "What does that mean?"

"Some of the nerves that come out from the brain stem have to do with this reflexive action of the eye, and apparently that's one of the areas that has damage."

The nurse practitioner adds,

"One of the things he'll need is followup with a neuro-ophthalmologist. Normally we see resolution of these problems over the course of a year. When Brian is discharged, we'll sit down and go over some of these things with you. You may find that your HMO is not real aware of the necessity for all the various kinds of followup that will be needed. We find the HMO's often don't know much about head injury."

The social worker says she has been in touch with Kaiser-Permanente. When Brian is considered medically stable, he will be transferred to Fairfax Hospital (15 minutes from our home). It will not be possible to transfer him directly to Mount Vernon, because Kaiser's doctors work only at Fairfax. Once he is at Fairfax, we will have additional discussions with them about rehabilitation. A copy of Brian's records will be sent to Mount Vernon Hospital so they can begin to assess the possibility of his admission there. We sign a form giving permission for the surgery and head back to Springfield.

Friday, August 23
When I arrive home from work, Curt looks anxious and explains that shock-trauma called. They did not take Brian in for surgery because they discovered an infection present in the meninges. We drive to

Baltimore feeling concerned, but only vaguely aware of the implications of this new development. We speak to Brad. He explains,

> "When I had my session with him early this morning, I noticed that his responses were poor. Just yesterday we had him on his feet and he took a few supported steps in the hall. We decided to do a spinal tap and found the infection."

The meninges are the three membranes that envelop the brain and spinal cord; Brian has cerebrospinal meningitis. Brad's eyes reflect anguish as he struggles to maintain some professional detachment, "It's in God's hands," he says.

Brian is back in the ICU, hooked up to the respirator; intravenous lines sprout from his arms; his eyes are bleary and inscrutable. Periodically, greenish fluid bubbles from his mouth and nose. I can't stand to look at him. I have no tears. The box of growing seeds and the box of demons are obliterated; near my heart is only a cold black void.

Sunday, August 25

I can't bear to see people and have to respond to their questions, "How is Brian doing?" I'm locked in "function" mode.

Monday, August 26

I go to work at Hogan & Hartson. Sarah, the secretarial coordinator, asks about Brian. I snap at her, "I don't want to talk about it."

Wednesday, August 28

The realization that death again hovers over Brian seeps into my mind. Up to this point I had not considered staying in Baltimore for extended periods, but now I must. I want to be there more constantly, to touch him, to minister to him, to be present to him. I learn of a nun in Baltimore, Sister Patricia O'Brien, whose convent might have an empty bed where I could stay for a few days. I call her. She sounds very kind and says of course I can stay with them at Bishop Keough convent, only 10 minutes from shock-trauma.

Saturday, August 31

I awake at 6:30 the next morning. Sister Patricia has fixed me bacon and eggs. I call the hospital and arrange to be there at one o'clock. I spend as much time with Brian as possible, massaging, applying a wet cloth to his forehead, talking in his ear, playing tapes: Bruce Springsteen, his grandparents' voices, the miracle stories from Matthew's gospel, and music that our folk group sings at Sunday Mass, "On Eagle's Wings."

> "He will raise you up on eagle's wings, bear you on the breath of dawn, make you to shine like the sun and hold you in the palm of his hand. You shall not fear the terror of the night, nor the arrow that flies by day. Upon his wings he will bear you up lest you dash your foot against a stone." (Joncas, *see References*) There is no discernible response.

That evening Sister Patricia, a social worker in a psychiatric hospital, takes me to dinner. She is a round, jolly Irish woman, and I take great pleasure in her companionship. I ask if she wants to come to the hospital with me –she is delighted to be asked. We stay with Brian for about an hour. He is having breathing spasms, like hiccups, that come and go periodically, but there is no response to our presence. She ties a scapular[3] on to his bed and we recite a prayer together. Sister Patricia kisses Brian on the cheek as we leave and says to him, "Here's a kiss from the fat Irish!"

Sister tells me on the way back to the convent that others in the Association of Christian Therapists tell her she has the gift of healing. She laughs at herself good-naturedly and tells me about one of her patients who was in intensive care,

> "I went to see her, prayed over her and she sat up in bed. She told me later, 'Why did you call me back. I was on my way down the road. I'd seen the others waiting for me, I wanted to go, and you called me back!'"

Monday, September 2

Seven weeks have passed since Brian's injury. I keep thinking, "I want to climb a mountain," partly for the physical release from the oppressions of shock trauma and partly because hiking in the Shenandoah Valley was a favorite recreation for Brian and his friends.

I ask Danny and two of his friends if they would like to go to see Skyline Caverns and hike on one of the trails. We emerge from the coolness of the caverns into intense heat and have lunch at one of the

---

3. An image of Jesus or Mary on a small piece of cloth attached to a cord, usually worn around the torso.

picnic tables. Then we find a two-mile trail and start up. Fifteen minutes later I start to feel dizzy. I sit down for a few seconds but do not listen to my body carefully. Within minutes, I pass out, falling down, but with no awareness of this event. In a few moments I stand up, seeing only Danny with me and trying to decide which fork of the trail to take. Danny looks distressed, and I have no idea why. Gradually it dawns on me that the other boys are missing. In the moments when I lost consciousness, they apparently decided on a very appropriate plan of action. Danny stayed with me while the others ran back down the trail for help.

I am still unaware of what has happened. Soon I see Chris and Steven coming up the trail with a ranger. He says, "The boys said a woman was hurt up here." I say absurdly but honestly, "I haven't seen anybody here!" The boys look at each other in wonderment and say to the ranger, "This is her." Then I see bruises on my legs and begin to realize what happened. The ranger escorts me back to his van to take my vital signs. An ambulance will come to take me to the local hospital for an examination.

I feel quite foolish, realizing I am the "comic relief" in this scenario. At the hospital I tell them I have been under stress and describe the events leading up to my passing out. It is decided that I probably had a mild hypoglycemic reaction, having eaten and rather quickly started a strenuous physical activity. They think it unwise that I attempt to drive back to Springfield and I agree. They will call Curt. "Please be sure to tell him I'm OK," I say, wondering how he will feel at being told his wife has been taken by ambulance to the Front Royal hospital. Our next door neighbors drive Curt down to pick us up and greet me with a smile, "It certainly is interesting living next to you folks!" Much later, I will realize that this loss of awareness of a few brief moments was a microscopic example of Brian's loss of a whole year of his life.

Wednesday, September 4

We meet again with Dr. Greenberg. The infection rages on in Brian's body, and fluid is building up in the ventricles of his brain. Another operation will be necessary. Just under the skin covering his skull they will place a shunt, a small tube that will allow the fluid to drain off into another part of his body.

> "The ventricle is like a blown up balloon at this point and the shunt will relieve pressure. There is a possibility that the tear will heal itself once pressure is relieved. This may also improve his responsiveness."

Friday, September 6

We see Brad in the hall and he says Brian responded to him by raising two fingers. He tells us his credibility is being questioned where Brian is concerned and that when testing Brian for response, he has to have a witness. His emotional involvement is well known around the unit. Dr. Garson, the handsome young intern on duty in ICU, smiles broadly and confirms the response that Brad saw.

Thursday, September 12

My sister Patty and her husband Roy are driving down from Pennsylvania to visit with me and Brian today. I am spending a few more days at the convent, and I take the bus to shock-trauma on this sunny, bright day with September crispness in the air.

When Patty and Roy arrive, Brian is fairly wakeful and attentive. The high point of the day is my request for him to "give me a finger." As I realize the double meaning of my request, I back-peddle, "Well, wait a minute, maybe I don't really want you to give me the finger!" A smile flickers across his face, ever so slight and ever so brief, but we all see it. The story of "the finger" spreads quickly around 4-D.

That evening I am alone with Brian in the ICU. Because the temperature is controlled in the ICU and because of all the lines connected to his body, Brian is covered only with a square cloth across his groin. He looks so whole, his body unmarked, his hair has begun to grow back; it is as if I could tear away the lines holding him and he would walk away with me. He seems like a young god, immobilized by forces he cannot master. Except for his feet, my eyes keep returning to his feet.

The hard skin on the soles of his feet is flaking away and I want to "fix" it. I mention my thoughts to Cada, the nurse on duty that night. She has a suggestion, "Let's make him some moon boots." She instructs me to rub lotion on his feet, then she sends me off to the microwave with absorbent pads we've wet under the faucet. We wrap the hot wet pads around his feet, finishing off with blue plastic coated pads, neatly wrapped, which do indeed look like moon boots!

Friday, September 13

Diane and Jack Jenc have invited us to go camping with them in the Shenandoah. Other friends will visit Brian in our absence. The autumn elegance of the Shenandoah Valley and congenial friendship make for a healing weekend. Around the campfire craziness, sing-alongs, boy scout skits—we get high on marshmallows.

Sunday, September 15

We hike up the Massanutten trail under sunny clear skies. Sitting near the top, enjoying the view, we watch a hawk soaring, close enough to count the feathers on his wing span.

Monday, September 16

I attend my first meeting of the N. Virginia Head Injury Foundation support group. As I haltingly describe what has happened to us since July 14, the details do not phase this group of people. They absorb my story gently, siphoning off some of the pain and tension. These are parents who've lived through very similar events and young men who were once as "hopeless" as Brian, not looking entirely whole, but walking, talking and telling their stories in engaging ways.

Tuesday, September 17

Curt and I and the children meet with Jerry and Bernice in Family Services. Bernice asks the children how things are different since Brian's accident. Eric says that things aren't too different, and I am utterly amazed that he can feel that way. I realize later that this is probably good –the disruption to their normal existence has not been too great at this point. It affirms our decision not to spend too much time at the hospital. We also discuss some faith issues. Bernice says, "Sometimes families ask, Why has God done this to us?" Scott's response is pragmatic, "Brian is in this condition because he hit a light pole in the middle of the night on the way to Ocean City; I don't think God had anything to do with it." I agreed with Scott's comment. Still... Why? and while I was on retreat! The Omni would have stayed in the driveway if I had been home! But this thinking feeds the demons, so I let it go and concentrate on a God who lights the way through dark passages.

The meningitis infection has subsided; they have removed the IV lines and the respirator. Brian's arms are as swollen and bruised as a junkie's.

Wednesday, September 18

We receive a call from Dr. Greenberg that the isotope scan reveals that the other tear in the membrane has indeed healed itself and Brian will not need the additional surgery. Good news, even if it is only plumbing! Teresa Robey, Brian's girlfriend from Longwood, who has been relaying messages to college friends, calls just after we receive this news, "All right! I gotta tell everyone in the dorm."

Thursday, September 19

The wiring is removed from Brian's jaw today, but he makes no attempt to open his mouth. I remember how I'd looked forward to this event, thinking he could then begin to speak and eat normally.

Tuesday, September 24

I decide to be at shock-trauma for the final hours before Brian's release and to ride back to Virginia with him in the ambulance. Curt drives me back to the convent that afternoon. A friend suggests taking a poster for everyone to sign for Brian, so we can read it to him when he wakes up. It is a good idea, as we are feeling acute withdrawal at this point, taking Brian away from all these people who know him.

Sister Patricia and I listen to a tape by Jean Vanier, who has established group homes for people with mental disabilities all over the world. As I talk with the sisters, I speak for the first time a latent thought, "It's almost as though we have to mourn the Brian who was as we gradually come to accept the Brian who is." How do we help that process for the whole family? A death might have been "easier." Dare I use such a casual word?

We have a final meeting with Brad, Dr. Menges (who performed the shunt surgery), Dr. Garson and Bernice Wolfson. I feel resentful and cynical about Dr. Greenberg's absence. The prognosis at this point is considerably less than his previous projections.

Brian is now being fed through a nasogastric tube; he is catheterized and the trach tube is still in place, mechanically suctioned regularly to keep his breathing passages open.

Brad tells us Brian is reacting consistently to pain stimulation only, pressure applied at the base of his fingernail. No one uses the word "coma" to describe Brian's present condition. We think of him as responding at Level II on the Rancho Los Amigos scale of recovery from coma, listed as "generalized response," defined as, "The patient is beginning to show signs of waking up. He reacts to deep pain (pinch). You may see the patient move around, open his eyes; however, he does not do this when asked."

After 73 days and $121,677, which has been totally covered by Kaiser-Permanente, Brian is now considered "medically stable" and ready to be moved to Fairfax Hospital, 15 minutes from our home.

The entry in my journal that night reflects graphically the confusion I felt: Final meeting. I am "holding up very well," they say. Once again, it is the neurosurgeon who must deliver the bad news. "There is irreversible damage to the brain stem," but at the end the qualifier, "but sometimes these patients surprise us." I remember Rose F. being told that her daughter would not reach an IQ above 50. I am walking a tightrope between reality and hope. I thank Dr. Menges for his help, ask if I can take everybody's picture and have them sign a poster for Brian when he wakes up. The angry demon in the box is raging as I perform this socially acceptable ritual. He wants to leap out and scream at the white-coated caricatures, "Maybe you should have let him die."

On the day Brian would have begun the fall semester at Virginia Tech, he and I enter the ambulance for the trip to Fairfax Hospital in Northern Virginia, Brian totally unaware of all that has happened to him and to us since July 14.

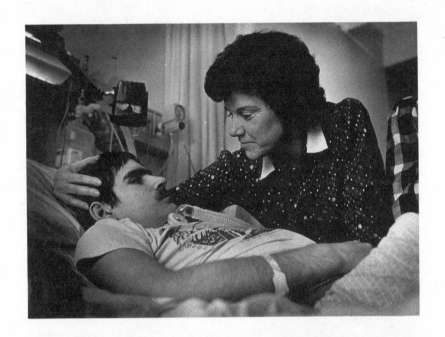

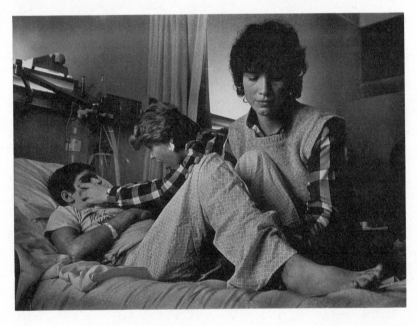

Brian in the Hospital. Photographs taken by The Washington Post (1985).

.2.

FROM WHENCE DOES
MY HELP COME

–Psalm 121

At the University of Maryland Hospital, we had listened, learned, observed and signed releases for surgery, with little questioning. The questions we had were unanswerable. What quality of life might Brian have? How far can he come back after two severe blows to his central nervous system? What parts of his brain are damaged? What *is* the prognosis?

At Fairfax Hospital, our role became one of advocacy as we realized the truth of the social worker's mild warning, "The HMO doctors may not know too much about head injury." Very little hope came from doctors who saw Brian at this stage. Our hope came from rekindled support and encouragement from our friends and faith community and from the mysterious power of prayers offered in our behalf. Additional support and information to help us grow as advocates came from people we met at meetings of the Northern Virginia Head Injury Foundation.

Hope also came from speech, physical, and occupational therapists who provided immediate continuity with Brad Swanson's work with Brian at shock-trauma. Irrepressible optimists, they went straight to work, undeterred by doctors who did not see the potential in Brian that they did.

This period marked the beginning of a struggle with systems still unresponsive to and unaware of the dimensions and possibilities of recovery from severe brain injury. It seemed to us that Kaiser's definition of rehabilitation was an extremely narrow one. Rehabilitation appeared among "Items Not Covered" in the basic policy brochure, along with "hearing aids," "experimental transplants," "plastic surgery." The spirit of rehabilitation we'd begun to understand was a great deal more than finishing touches, rather the difference between a person

who is responsive to his environment and one who is not, hardly in the
same category as plastic surgery. We knew that Kaiser Permanente's
policy did not cover admittance to a rehabilitation facility, estimated at
$18,000 a month, but, had put this problem on hold while Brian
struggled to survive the meningitis infection.

As we tried to grasp what options we might have, Curt called the
U. S. Office of Personnel Management, which administers the health
insurance plans for federal employees, asking for a clearer contractual
definition of "rehabilitation." No government definition existed; Kaiser's
23–page brochure contained everything we were entitled to as subscribers. I also obtained a legal opinion from a Hogan & Hartson attorney and
learned we had no legal recourse.

Curt and I had talked about the possibility of mortgaging our
$180,000 house or my going to work full time as ways we could pay for
Brian's rehabilitative care. Friends also suggested setting up a trust fund
for neighborhood contributions. But the money we could raise from
these actions would barely touch the surface, and no one could tell us
how long Brian might need rehabilitative care. We continued to believe
there was some room for compromise with Kaiser; perhaps they would
pay for half of Brian's care at a facility like Mount Vernon Hospital or
at least an amount comparable to what they were willing to pay if he
were placed in a nursing home.

My first visit with Pat D. of Kaiser Permanente, a former nurse
assigned to Brian's case, took place in a small meeting room at Fairfax
Hospital. In response to my questions along the above lines, Pat's
answer was simple and unbending, "No." We were grateful that Brian's
already enormous bill was completely covered by Kaiser Permanente,
but it seemed unthinkable that they would drop us in the middle of the
process. It was a catch-22 of the classic sort; if Brian's responses
improved, making him eligible for rehabilitation, our funds would be
cut off. If he was placed in a nursing home, depressing as that thought
was, at least we would not be facing immediate financial disaster, since
100 days of care in such a facility would be covered by Kaiser.

THE DOCTORS

The second day at Fairfax I met Dr. H., the first Kaiser doctor to
examine Brian. She listened carefully to my observations concerning
the thorazine prescribed at shock-trauma to control Brian's breathing

spasms. I had researched this drug and discovered that his lack of responsiveness could be a side effect. She quickly agreed to discontinue the medication since it was having no effect on the spasms. I was pleased to have established a working relationship with "Brian's doctor."

At the beginning of the next week, I discovered, to my dismay, that a different Kaiser doctor would be making the rounds at Fairfax each week.

I met Dr. S., the doctor of the week. After her examination, she and I walked into a nearby waiting room to talk.

"You've been through quite an ordeal, haven't you, "she began sympathetically. "It's very difficult," I said, "with all this modern medical technology, we're creating a new group of survivors, but we don't have the proper services in place to bring them back to a meaningful existence."

Dr. S. took the conversation down a different track. She told me about premature babies who were being "saved," mentioning a particular hospital in Massachusetts, then placed in nursing homes. "At least you've had Brian for twenty years, but how could anyone visit a preemie in a nursing home and have feeling for life at such a limited level."

The next phase of the conversation is hazy in my memory, but by some progression of thoughts, she was saying, "Maybe if he were to get another infection, we ought to consider withholding treatment." I probably nodded meekly in agreement.

My internal wanderings on death as a more merciful fate than a severely limited life had been spoken to no one, only written in my personal journal. Ethical considerations about continued treatment were never discussed by professionals at shock-trauma.

Rita Buesgens, the social worker, had already met me for a brief intake interview. After Dr. S. left the meeting room, I headed distractedly to Rita's office, wandering in a gray quagmire between the box of hopeful seeds and the box of demons. I mumbled tearfully to her, "I don't know if I'm angry with her, or grateful that the subject is at least out in the open." What if, what if! I couldn't imagine having to make such a decision and where we would go for support and wise counsel.

I discussed the conversation with Curt that evening and we decided that I would visit Barbara Mishkin, another Hogan & Hartson attorney who works in medical ethics. Curt and I were unable to discuss the deeper implications of the question.

Tuesday, October 1

I visit Barbara Mishkin in her office. She says, "If it were my son, and I were faced with such a decision, I would want him examined by Dr. Ayub Ommaya. He used to be at National Institute of Health (NIH), and he's very knowledgeable. Here's his phone number; I'm sure he'd be happy to come and examine him." She also gives me the name of a priest at Georgetown University, a Catholic ethicist. I am buoyed with new hope and a new name and put in a call to Ommaya's office immediately.

During the course of the day, my benign feelings about Dr. S. have turned to smoldering anger, as I consider the entire context of our conversation. She represents the organization paying the bills, and she has seen Brian only once. Just looking over his charts, already an imposing stack of data, how could she begin to understand all the effort, the professional caring, the ups and downs of our experience since July 14! Curt too has had a conversation with her during the day. He says quietly, "She didn't sound very hopeful." I think about Dr. S. that night, mostly in a calm manner. Curt and I agree that we wanted her off the case; we have been advised that we have that option with any particular doctor. I plan to speak with her the next day, as carefully and firmly as possible, and point out that I feel we misunderstood one another in our earlier conversation. I believe that this communication can take place in a business-like way without my anger bursting from the box in full flame, reducing me to "a hysterical mother."

Wednesday, October 2

I go again to the hospital. Brian's color is gray. An unexplained indentation at his left temple looks more pronounced than I'd ever seen it. He is not responding to any stimulus. He looks as if he is dying, and I become acutely aware that the person in charge may be looking for signs to discontinue treatment. I put in another call from the hospital to Dr. Ommaya's office to ask that he call me at the number in Brian's room.

While Dr. S. is examining Brian during her rounds for the day, and before I've had a chance to speak with her, Dr. Ommaya calls. "Yes, I will be glad to examine Brian, but I will need his doctor to make a note in the chart, since I do not have visiting doctor's privileges at Fairfax Hospital." I tell him I will get that permission and call him back. I am blunt with Dr. S., "That was Doctor Ayub Ommaya, a doctor I want to examine Brian. I need you to make a note in his chart to that effect."

She becomes defensive, "I can't do that without knowing who he is. What kind of doctor is he, a neurologist?" Unfortunately I don't know, I only know that I respect Barbara Mishkin and that Dr. Ommaya has a national reputation. By this time all opportunity for measured conversation between Dr. S. and myself has evaporated. I shoot back, "He's very famous and I want him to see Brian!" She stalks out of the room, saying something about not having time for this. I say I will get the necessary information and write it out for her before she leaves the floor. In a few minutes I hand her a slip of paper with his name, address, phone number and the fact that he is a neurosurgeon.

On the way home, I stop at the library to look him up in Who's Who. I find that he studied at Oxford University in England, began as a visiting scientist at NIH in 1963, progressing to associate neurosurgeon 1963-68, on to chief of neurosurgery in 1974-79. We learn the next day that Kaiser has approved Ommaya's consult and will pay his fee.

Tuesday, October 8

Dr. Ayub Ommaya has just examined Brian, using a technique called a cold caloric which involves squirting ice water into Brian's ear canal, then watching for reactions. I am sitting now with Dr. Ommaya in the waiting room, having obtained his permission to tape our conversation.

"Well," he begins in a measured, accented tone, "going through the records and looking at him now I see that he had a very severe head injury. The additional unfortunate thing was the severe infection. Initially it was treated without a culture. They used a broad spectrum of antibiotics and never really got good control of it. With a heavy meningitis infection, the bacteria consume a lot of oxygen, depriving the brain cells of needed oxygen. This additional deprivation of oxygen from the brain is like a stroke on top of a head injury.

"The ice water test I did is for stimulating the brain stem, the core of the brain. The eyeballs should move. There was no movement at all. It was fixed, rigid. No response at all from the left side and minimal response from the right, indicating that the brain stem is almost totally wiped out. Response to pain is also limited, reflexive rather than purposeful. This is now the third month. When patients like this have a positive caloric test, there is some hope of a reconnection. But if the stem responses don't return, then I'm afraid the chances are not very good."

"Would you repeat that again," I say shakily.

"If there is no change in his response to the ice water test, the chances of his waking up are nil," Ommaya replies.

"But," I say, gathering confidence, "another mother told me that even though part of the brain stem is damaged, by constantly working with a patient, those neurons can reconnect. Under certain conditions, that does happen, right?"

"It happens if you have a working brain stem. The part that controls blood pressure and heart rate is working, but connections to the higher part of the brain are not working. So at this moment it doesn't look very good, I'm afraid. The caloric test should be tried again over the next few weeks. You are reaching a point where you will have to make a decision in terms of care."

"Yes," I respond, "and we are having a hard time with that. We've met people who have recovered even though doctors have said there's nothing there! It's very hard to think of putting him in a nursing home. We've seen Brian fight for his life through each crisis and we just feel that the Kaiser doctors are too willing to give up on him after only a week of observation!"

"Yes, I understand," he replies, "it is a very major decision you have to make and you need more objective data. I will also recommend evoke potential tests to see what information is being processed. If there is no change within the next three to four weeks, you will probably have to find another place for him."

I try another path, "You were formerly affiliated with NIH; is there any kind of research program available that we might get him into?"

Now I hear Dr. Ommaya's concerns, "No, I started something when I was there, but it was very hard to get support because we were highly experimental. At the moment there is no interest in head injury. The young population is the most affected and NIH is not interested. It is very frustrating."

I mention to Dr. Ommaya that Dr. Bortnik, a neurosurgeon at Fairfax, is going to operate on Brian this week to move the shunt from the lung to the stomach because he is having a continuing buildup of fluid in his lungs.

"Good," Dr. Ommaya approves, "pleural shunts don't work very well. Most people are doing peritoneal shunts where the tube runs into the tummy. In the old days when the shunts were developing they tried all kinds of placements, but the consensus all over the world is that the peritoneal is the best."

Anger flashes through me–*why* didn't they do it right at shock-trauma, and *why* didn't they "get control" of the meningitis sooner? Does anyone know what they are doing?

When we finish our conversation, we shake hands. I thank him and feel some ego satisfaction with the quality of my "interview." Fifteen minutes later when I reach my car alone, I weep uncontrollably and I wonder what happened to Barbara Wawa, the interviewer. She's gone. An emotionally ragged mother is back.

During the next day, the energies from the box gradually transform; no longer demons, they become the forces of life–courage, determination. I will not give Brian over to death, or a living death, without a fight!

Thursday, October 10

The first challenge is to convince Kaiser there are good reasons to authorize a few more weeks of the full range of therapies provided by Fairfax Hospital. I awaken this morning, combative and determined, as we prepare for a meeting at the hospital with Pat D. and two doctors from Kaiser Permanente, Dr. M., a pediatrician, and Dr. R., internal medicine, who had phone contact with shock-trauma doctors during Brian's care in Baltimore.

In addition to the three Kaiser representatives present is the social worker, who has offered to sit in for moral support. She agrees that we will be under pressure to move him to a nursing home very soon.

After some preliminary greetings, Dr. R. says Brian is in a coma, like Karen Quinlan. The reference shocks me; as yet, the word "coma" had not been used by a professional speaking to us since the meningitis infection. We thought of coma as no response. In our newly learned framework, Brian *was* responding occasionally on the second level of the Rancho los Amigos scale. I mention the Rancho scale and Dr. R. looks puzzled. I suggest not too kindly that he ought to do his homework. Dr. M. mentions "code decisions," apparently referring to the question of taking extraordinary measures to save him if he gets another infection. We are given no context in which to consider this question. We reply with conviction that for now at least, we want everything possible done for him.

In an effort to inject a little humanity into this bloodless meeting,

I read from a note Brian's friend Teresa had written after her visit with him yesterday,

> "He squeezed my hand quite a bit and moved fingers and toes. He played tug of war with a washcloth. He arm wrestled a little. He put pretty much into it too. When I told him I had to go, he shook his head and wouldn't let go of my hand."

Pat D. says a bed is available at a nursing home in Manassas, and we are fortunate, since often there is a waiting list for such accommodations. We ignore that point and discuss the incongruity of Kaiser's policy not to cover rehabilitation if Brian becomes eligible. Dr. M. agrees this is probably not a good policy, "but speaking to us about it will not help, we are just doctors." He says that writing an appeal to Kaiser management would certainly be appropriate.

After this discussion, the two doctors accompany us to Brian's room, where speech therapist Debi Gale has agreed to meet us and work with Brian briefly to demonstrate the generalized response she has seen. Dr. R. looks carefully and does indeed notice that Brian is tracking movement with his eyes. We discuss Dr. Ommaya's recommendations, and they agree that a few more weeks at Fairfax would be appropriate. We end the meeting not too cordially, but feeling satisfied with this small victory–we've bought a little more time.

That afternoon I go to the library and look up articles on Karen Quinlan. I read that her father visited her every day in a nursing home for ten years till she finally died, her body shrunken and atrophied. During that time she occasionally responded to him with a smile or eye movement, but that was all.

The next day I move my desk and typewriter into a small upstairs bedroom and rap out an angry two-page letter to Kaiser management, describing the impossible position we find ourselves in because of their lack of coverage in such a catastrophic case as Brian's.

THE STATE OF MARYLAND

A couple days after this meeting, a bill arrived from the State of Maryland, addressed to me: "Damage to a utility pole on Route 50, caused by car bearing license plate MSRIFE. Please remit $762.00." I raged, out of control, declaring they could take me to the highest court, I would not pay for their stupid pole! Curt, whose stoicism was sometimes comforting and at other times exasperating, pointed out after tolerating my hysteria for some time, that our auto insurance would pay this bill. Still, the absurdity held me, insurance to pay for the light pole, but no insurance to pay for Brian's rehabilitation!

LEVEL III

Spurred on to new creativity by Teresa's reports, I bring some props with me one evening. We are looking for response that corresponds to Level III on the Rancho los Amigos scale -localized response, being able to follow simple directions: close your eyes, turn your head, squeeze my hand, let go of my hand. I have a favorite T-shirt with me this evening; Mark Holland had referred to it in pictures from the dorm "Brian in his damn Tarheels shirt." He reacts strongly to it, reaching out with his hand. I also brought a banana and some peanut butter in a small cup since reaction to familiar smells would also indicate that the message is at least getting through the brain stem. He closes his hand around the banana, but the peanut butter he ignores.

He looks alert, so I try talking to him about learning to eat again, "It would be great to help you eat some real food." (And get rid of that invasive tube stuck up your nose!) Having decided I want Brian to live, my hope for the quality of his life begins to focus on two specific issues–communication and eating. More advanced hopes can remain on hold while we pray and work toward these two primary breakthroughs.

I show him a picture of the brain from a Washington Post article about four–year–old Maranda, half of whose brain was removed as treatment for a seizure disorder. The areas of the cerebral cortex are outlined in color, the sensory region, the regions that control body motion, intellect, behavior, reading and writing. The article reports that Maranda's right hemisphere is doing a remarkable job of taking over most of her body functions.

I explain to him that he has had an injury to the brain stem. "Brian, you are not paralyzed. You must try to move various parts of your body upon request, to reconnect the circuits." His expression is inscrutable. I get out the drawing board that Karen brought for him. I put the pen in his hand and try to duplicate Brad's work with him many weeks ago. We write his name B R I A N. I think perhaps he cooperated, but I am hardly a scientific observer, just a mom trying to fertilize the seeds of hope.

Another way to nourish that hope was to again encourage friends to help us call Brian back. Now three months since his injury, only a few people were still involved, but a specific request for help might rekindle the energies of community and church.

After we explained the need, this note appeared in the Cursillo[4] newsletter:

> *"As many of you know, Brian Rife has been hospitalized since July. Prayers for him and his family are important and needed. As part of Brian's rehabilitation there is a continuing request for visitors to stimulate him in conversation, reading, playing music; to let Brian know of our presence and that it is important for him and us that he return to our community. If you find it fits in your spiritual journey, perhaps you could journey to Fairfax Hospital to spend time with Brian and Jesus (you'll find both of them there)."*

Within a few days, people were newly aware of our dilemma and began responding to our requests for additional visitors for Brian, to provide as much stimulation as possible during the coming crucial weeks. I wrote up a poster for his room that read:

> *Brian is usually able to respond to visitors in a general way. Speak to him in a clear positive voice, tell him who you are. He will usually open his eyes. If not, don't give up too easily. Ice water and a washcloth are available at the nurse's desk. Speak clearly about what you are doing:*

> *"Brian, I'm wiping your forehead with a cold cloth."*
> *"Brian, I'm going to say a prayer with you."*
> *"Brian, I'm going to move your arm to exercise it a bit." (see instructions from physical therapist on wall about range of motion exercises.) If he is wakeful, reading from Louis L'Amour (his favorite author) is a possibility.*

> *Assume That He Hears You!*

> *We are looking especially for localized responses, such as moving a hand or foot in response to a request, or reaching out to touch an object presented to him. There is a small note book in the drawer. Please note your visit and any particular reaction you observed.*

4. The Cursillo is a short course in Christian living; now worldwide and ecumenical, it began in Spain in 1947.

Some of the most helpful visitors were those who had "been there." John and Joan Verna, having struggled together during John's long rehabilitation from a stroke, spoke to Brian with strong confidence, born of their experience, "Let's see a thumbs up, Brian, you're looking good, you're going to be all right." Brian responded with his eyes and lifted his thumb. Joan told me privately, "Don't listen to the neurosurgeons, they're always so negative!"

GOING PUBLIC

In early October, we took another action that proved significant. As the dimensions of the insurance issue became clear, I thought of enlisting the help of the news media but was hesitant about inviting a reporter into our lives in the midst of such a personal crisis. But the idea was affirmed by a neighbor and by Sister Patricia in Baltimore during one of my conversations with her.

Two years earlier, I'd met a writer at The Washington Post named Neil Henry. Neil had written a powerfully moving front-page series on migrant workers during a time when I was enrolled in a journalism course at Trinity College in Washington. I interviewed him for an assignment but had not spoken with him since that time. I considered him to be a sensitive person and I admired his talent. During the first week of Brian's stay at Fairfax Hospital, I called Neil and asked for his help. He expressed his sympathy, but only a marginal interest in the story until after several conversations with us and a visit with Brian at the hospital. "It's quite a different thing, seeing him and just hearing about him," he said. I passed on to him information from the Head Injury Foundation, the only national organization involved in advocacy for survivors of brain injury, and gradually he saw our story as representative of a much larger problem.

After our meeting with Kaiser Permanente personnel, the details of which we spilled out to him on the phone that evening, Neil attended a meeting of the N. Virginia Head Injury Foundation with us and heard stories from families whose relatives remained at a low level of consciousness. Bill H. spoke about the process of finding a nursing home for his son when he did not come out of the coma, "Some of the places I visited weren't fit for a dog. He's at Leesburg Memorial Hospital now. At least it's not all geriatric patients, and they give him some therapy." Neil wanted to accompany us if we began to visit nursing homes.

That meeting fed my worst fears of what could happen. The note in my journal reflects a swing backwards:

I am angry and isolated, cutting off friends who are trying so hard to help, who tell me I "must have hope." The only phrasing that makes sense is from Bill H., "You don't give up hope, but you do have to adjust your expectations." I don't know where to focus the anger; I hate shock-trauma and their medical "miracles"! I feel guilty because I'm agreeing with Dr. S. that life in such a ruined state may not be worth living. I am awake most of the night–night terrors–court cases for the right to allow someone to die. After four years, Bill's son still smiles occasionally. How eerie, how emotionally impossible! He is there, but he is not there. The only prayer I can form is "My God, why have you forsaken me?"

THE HIGH PLACES

We have received countless letters of support and encouragement since the day of Brian's accident, but one stands out. Don Resset, a friend in Montana, whose 42-year-old wife died tragically the previous year, wrote, several weeks after I'd written him about Brian's accident:

Dear Curt and Janet,

I've hoped and prayed that the Lord will restore Brian to wholeness but also that He will give you strength and courage to face what is happening to each of you in this situation. I've started letters several times but each time I stopped, knowing the words weren't coming as I knew they should.

Then last week I went to visit a couple who had lost a 21 –year–old son last June to an asthma attack. They had a terrible time with his death and still are, but we talked about not the why of tragedy but the how. How are we going to change tragedy to triumph? Are we going to make life more meaningful, are we going to love more deeply, are we going to be more patient, are we going to be more compassionate, are we going to appreciate those around us more, are we going to make life for the living better because we care?

Or will we be bitter, self-centered individuals who can only see that God did us wrong. I don't think so. I don't think a loving compassionate God, who wept at the tomb of Lazarus, has anything to do with death, tragedy and suffering. I think those are all products of an imperfect world, made imperfect by sin. And just as God limits His power to allow us freedom of choice so too does He limit His power in the area of suffering. He weeps with us when we weep, just as we weep for our children when they are hurt.

There is a verse in Isaiah, "They that hope in the Lord shall renew their strength, they shall take wings as eagles." The eagle has some interesting characteristics –when a storm approaches the eagle doesn't bed down in shelter but finds the highest point around and there he waits for the storm and he faces into it and begins flying. The harder the winds blow, the higher the eagle soars. Let suffering take you to new heights of compassion and love.

HOPEFUL SIGNS

Towards the end of October, we began to receive encouraging notes from therapists. From Debi Gale, speech therapist:

"I spent a long time with Brian early this morning. He was relatively easily aroused repeatedly by a variety of moderate stimuli, plus a lot of reflexive responses. Solidly level 2 on Rancho scale at this point."

From Johanna Brady, occupational therapist:

"We want to let you know that we have seen some lovely changes in Brian. He has been tracking with his eyes, smiling, and raised his right hand three times to verbal command. We had him upstairs working on the mat and were able to place him in multi-positions. He tolerated all this very well and was thoroughly fatigued at the end of one hour and a half. We are rooting for him all the way."

At the end of October, Dr. Roger Gisolfi, the physiatrist from Mount Vernon Hospital, agrees to see Brian again. He had examined him briefly at Kaiser's request just after we arrived at Fairfax Hospital. He is also aware by this time that a <u>Post</u> reporter is involved in our case.

I've asked Brian's friend, Jack Winstead, who had lent us his car back in July, to be present this morning to assist in eliciting response from Brian, since it is so important that we convince Dr. Gisolfi he is a good candidate for Mount Vernon's rehabilitation program. We try to wake him up without much success, Jack slapping his arm saying, "C'mon, Brian!" When Dr. Gisolfi strides in, with an assistant in tow, we renew our efforts. Brian remains still. But Dr. G. brushes our effort aside, "I don't have to see firsthand, I've seen the therapists' notes. I will call Dr. R. at Kaiser and let him know we'll take Brian as a rehab patient." It's surely the best news we've had in weeks!

On November 19, we finally receive word that Kaiser Permanente has reconsidered and will fund Brian's care at Mount Vernon Hospital for 60 days. No coincidence that as Neil had interviewed Kaiser management about our case, radio ads were broadcast, soliciting new subscribers with a promise of "total care."

THE NOTEBOOK

Meanwhile, dozens of entries have been made in the little yellow spiral notebook by Brian's visitors. A few of them:

10/14/85   Brian was very tired –moved his fingers on command several times. Moved his hand towards mine when I asked him to. Also moved muscles in his face (left side) twice. I also asked Brian to hold the seashell and squeeze it. He held it on his own and did the same with his blue shirt.

—Sue

10/24   Mrs. Winstead & I arrived at the same time. Two of Brian's physical therapists were here working with him. They felt he had better "range of motion" today. Also said by next week they would be working with him in the therapy room upstairs. Two smiles this afternoon for me. Fantastic response when Jack walked in. A big smile and one finger shot up and good expression. Note: first time I've seen Brian's lips open.

—Sharon

10/29   This is the best I've seen Brian in a long time. Very alert for an hour. Looked at the family pictures –eyes moved from one picture to the next. Smiled at the graduation picture (with Karen). Responded with "pain" as he was receiving a new IV line. More smiles when I showed him my new glasses. When the therapist told him to wave to me, he slightly raised three fingers.

—Sharon

10/23   Frank Beto and I visited Brian. I could not rouse him very much. We talked and patted his left hand. Applied some ice to his neck with little reaction. We talked some more and left him with Bruce Springsteen on the tape recorder. Love,

—Pete H.

10/26   Half awake when I arrived. Opened eyes –good expression on face; a couple of smiles when doing arm exercises (with jokes). Eyes look better. Doesn't like to have his fanny rubbed.

—Sharon

11/2   Brian slept the whole time. I could only get him to wake up for a few minutes.

—Sue W.

11/6   Brian is very sleepy today. Had a busy morning –down to X-ray, etc. Eyes half open but not too responsive.

—Sharon and Linda Krebs

11/8   Brian was sleepy. Opened his eyes when I talked to him but kept closing them.

—Diane Jenc

OUR FAMILY

Through all the focus on Brian, we tried to keep some normalcy in our family life, but it was not easy. His condition and events surrounding him absorbed an enormous amount of Curt's and my energy. We did alert counselors at the schools Danny and Eric attended about the ongoing crisis in the family, so they might be aware of effects it had on the boys. We encouraged Eric, Danny and Sheri to accompany us to the hospital, but they were often resistant. The boys' relationship with Brian had been a very physical one, playing frisbee and basketball when he came home from college. Sheri, only 18 months younger than Brian, saw him as her favorite confidante in the family. Confined to a hospital bed, unable to respond to them, this new Brian was not someone they were anxious to see, but they tried and gradually became more aware of what had happened to him, how it was affecting all of us, and why we had to keep working to help Brian respond.

We mused that if Brian had been in college, we would have seen very little of him that fall, perhaps an occasional phone call or a letter requesting a bit more spending money!

One evening, Danny and Eric accompanied us. Eric seemed very tuned in, talking to Brian with more ease than at any previous time, but Danny appeared troubled, unable to get too close, almost claustrophobic. I tuned in to Danny's confusion and found myself equally unable to reach out to Brian. Danny and I went on a tour of the hospital, checking out the cafeteria, coke and candy machines. I overcompensated, spending $8.50 on ice cream, gummy fish and chocolate-covered peanuts.

On Halloween night, I went trick-or-treating with Danny and his friend Chris, then took Danny in his costume to the hospital to visit Brian. Danny seemed more comfortable this visit, but after ten minutes, it was time to go home.

Other nights, I resisted going to the hospital myself, feeling like I was losing touch with my other children. One evening the house seemed so full of chaos, children loud and unruly, I was aware I went to see Brian because he was the only one who wouldn't talk back!

One place I seemed most able to forget Brian for a while was at the soccer field. It was a particular joy that fall watching Danny and Eric in their bright colored jerseys, their hair blowing in the wind. Both excellent players, their healthy bodies moved expertly around the field, and I found myself cheering with complete abandon when either of them made a well-executed play.

On Thanksgiving Day, we made a tape of our family conversation at dinner and Curt, his parents, and Scott, home from Virginia Tech for the holiday, took it with them to the hospital in the evening. I stayed home to play Tripoli with the younger boys.

The day after Thanksgiving, Mark Holland, Brian's old dorm friend, visited. That night, the whole family enjoyed dinner at a restaurant to celebrate Sheri's 19th birthday, with Mark accompanying us. It was like having a surrogate "big brother" present. He shared dorm stories with us, a few too many beer blasts perhaps, but Mark's southern Virginia charm and easy manner was good for all of us. We stopped by the hospital afterwards and sang Happy Birthday to Sheri with Brian. His response was limited and Sheri left the room in tears. But she tried again in a few days, this time more encouraged by his alertness and appearance, after a haircut and a new T-shirt.

DELAYS

Brian was supposed to be moved to Mount Vernon the end of November, but there is a delay. The Kaiser doctors, now more aware of Brian's needs, have decided to surgically place a feeding tube directly into his stomach, allowing him to be nourished more efficiently than with the nasogastric tube. He weighs 125 pounds, 20 pounds less than before the accident. It is likely to be a long time before Brian can eat normally.

Difficulties develop with the placement of the tube and until it is functioning properly, he will not be transferred.

One afternoon when Mark and I visit the hospital, we enter the room to find that the Kaiser ophthalmologist had ordered both of his eyes patched, closing out all outside stimulus. She has legitimate concerns about the condition of his corneas, but no one has discussed the decision with us. Annoyed, I impulsively remove the patches, understandably upsetting the head nurse. The "on-duty" nurses are emotionally sympathetic to my action, if not professionally so. Too many people treating so many different parts of Brian, but who is looking at the whole Brian? I am anxious to have him moved to Mount Vernon where Dr. Gisolfi will provide this much needed oversight.

I discuss my frustration over the delay with Dr. Gisolfi, who tells me to relax, "It buys us a little more time." Sixty days of funding is in fact a very short time when it comes to brain injury rehabilitation. He also advises me to follow the ophthalmologist's recommendations about Brian's eyes. I'm learning to choose my issues more carefully.

LEVEL IV

On November 21st, I arrive at the hospital to observe Debi's session with him. Brian is highly agitated. He has thrown up and the nurses are cleaning up. His level of awareness is high, his breathing stressed and his expression one of "what is going on?" The nurses and I speak to calm him. When Debi comes in she decides not to do her usual session, but does get out the earphones that help him to focus on the single sound of her voice. He reaches up very purposefully, grabbing the earphone, clearly indicating "I don't want this on my head!" by his gesture. We both praise him for the communication and remove the earphones. When I am alone with him, I sense a real desire to speak. Today Brian's responses correspond to Level IV on the Rancho scale, defined as confused-agitated.

INSIGHTS

That same week, I recorded a dream in my journal:

I am in the hallway at the hospital with two friends. Brian's bed is in the hallway; somehow he is out of it and standing against the wall, propped up. I notice and shout for help, "He can't stand alone–help me get him back in bed!" Then we are in a different room, moving him from one bed to his regular bed. In the process, his head is bumped and he cries, like a baby, a loud wail. I embrace him to comfort him and he hugs me back, a good strong hug, like that of the "real" Brian. I tell him how good that feels and he laughs–it is again the laugh of a baby.

I learned later that Brian's friend Karen had a dream with strikingly similar images. We decided as we explored these dreams that they reflected our subconscious anxiety about what might come next.

The next meeting of the Head Injury Foundation was led by Dr. Peter Patrick, a neuropsychologist at Mount Vernon Hospital. Discussing family issues in a straightforward manner, he said:

> "Families can get stuck in perpetual vigilance, feeling that they must be present at all times, anxious and worried. They can come to think of the injured person as so special and a 'miracle recovery' that it becomes very difficult to reintegrate the person realistically into the family after a long rehabilitation process."

Dr. Patrick also clarified behavioral issues during the rehabilitation process: physical and verbal loss of inhibitions, disruption of sexuality, poor orientation to reality. Neil, who had accompanied us again, leaned over to me at one point saying, "Doesn't this scare you?" I replied that it did not because I'd been aware of many of these things since my early conversation with Rose F. Hearing them again was helping me to integrate the information.

Relating an experience in his own family, Dr. Patrick talked about the denial mechanism. He and his wife, a registered nurse, have a son who has epilepsy. "We were filling out a school medical form for him," he said, "and he just had two grand mal seizures." When we saw epilepsy on the form, my wife looked at me and said, "Does he have epilepsy?"

Dr. Patrick also pointed out that night, with considerable frustration, "The neurosurgeons are always saying 'He won't make it,' when in fact 85-90 per cent do survive at this point."

The next day, I felt more awareness of the "denial" issue. Perhaps my recent swing back to dwelling on the possibility of Brian's death was a form of denial and unwillingness to walk the long, tedious path ahead. By mid-November it seemed firmer in my mind that Brian was not going to die. We would go on through the process that lay ahead of us and we would survive!

THE PEOPLE OF GOD

From the beginning, our faith community helped us, with hearts, hands, minds and prayers. When we left for that first drive to Baltimore, the members of my spiritual support group acted concretely in ways that expressed their individuality, Pat tucking a $20 bill in my pocket, Joan handing me two Valium pills and Rosalie bringing her well-thumbed Bible. During the weeks that followed, Rosalie became my most sensitive spiritual friend, a "priest" who listened patiently to my despairs, but called me gently to faith and hope.

Days after the accident, friends served as a message center to take calls and pass on information about Brian's progress. We asked people not to call those first few weeks, but notes and cards were welcome. These notes were read aloud to the entire family so that everyone could experience this sense of support from friends, neighbors and Curt's fellow Amway distributors. Dozens of cards and letters arrived, along with an enormous supply of food: ham, potato salad, roast beef, cakes and pies, a pot of chili. Originally the plan was to coordinate meals as well, but eventually we just let everything come and used our large freezer for storage. Weeks passed before we consumed all the food. Some notes included cash, "to pay for gas for trips to Baltimore." Many offered to make the trip with us, day or evening, according to their availability. It was difficult, especially for Curt, to accept this kind of help, but the realization of our physical and emotional limitations made us increasingly receptive and grateful.

We had written to our extended community around the country, Brian's godparents in California, friends in South Dakota and Montana, and were assured of the prayer support of many spiritual communities. The endless variety of expressions and actions created a beautiful mosaic of the "people of God," from the spiritually sublime–Rhoda Nary and her husband traveling in England saying a special prayer for Brian and for all of us in each of the cathedrals they visited–to the down-to-earth practical–Linda Hardin offering free haircuts for the whole family and John Guarino's offer of a free therapeutic massage for Curt and myself. Neighbor Sharon Crandall, something of a second mother to Brian over the years since Brian and her daughter Karen were infants, was a helpful friend and hospital visitor, making frequent entries in our notebook at Fairfax.

Many others responded to the call for visitors for Brian, faithfully noting their observations. Women friends were especially present to me many times, aware when I wanted to "talk about it" and when I wanted to talk about almost anything else. Their ability to "shift gears" at an instant's notice was uncanny. We planned a Mass to celebrate and affirm this magnificent variety.

Approximately sixty people gathered in our living room the evening of December 6, with Father Paul Wynants as celebrant. Guitarists and singers from the parish folk group provided the music.

After greetings to the group gathered, not all of whom knew each other, and an expression of the inter-relatedness of all their prayers and actions, I explained our reasons for choosing the responsorial psalm, "We thank you, God, for the wonder of our being."

"We take so many things for granted, the miracle of our minds as the message center of our bodies, the seat of our consciousness, of who we are. We have experienced graphically the damage a moment's impact can have on that delicate system."

For the first reading and the responsorial we had chosen Psalm 139. John Verna read, his voice breaking:

> *Truly you have formed my inmost being;*
> *you knit me in my mother's womb.*
> *I give thanks that I am fearfully, wonderfully made;*
> *wonderful are your works.*
>
> *My soul also you knew full well;*
> *nor was my frame unknown to you*
> *When I was made in secret,*
> *when I was fashioned in the depths of the earth.*

The response flowed powerfully,

> *"We thank you God for the wonder of our being."*

The second reading from 1 Corinthians, Chapter 12:

> *There are different gifts but the same Spirit, there are different*
> *ministries but the same Lord. The body is one and has many*
> *members, many though they are, are one body; and so it is with*
> *Christ. It was in one Spirit that all of us, whether Jew or Greek,*
> *slave or free, were baptized into one body... As it is, God has set*
> *each member of the body in the place he wanted it to be... that there*
> *may be no dissension in the body, but that all the members may be*

concerned for one another. If one member suffers, all the members suffer with it; if one member is honored, all the members share its joy. You, then, are the body of Christ.

Father Paul read from the Gospel of John, Chapter 15:

I am the true vine
and my father is the vinegrower.
He prunes away every barren branch
but the fruitful ones he trims clean
to increase their yield...
Live on in me, as I do in you...
I am the vine, you are the branches.

When we sang, "Lay your hands gently upon us, let their touch render your peace, let them bring your forgiveness and healing, lay your hands, gently lay your hands,"(Landry) we were pleading for healing for all of us, not only Brian. We were mothers and fathers, husbands and wives, sons and daughters, all broken or hurt in one way or another, merely by the fact of our existence. But within that gathering we drew strength and hope from one another and from the spirit of Jesus Christ.

In front of our living room couch sits a round stone table etched with drawings from the 12th century Bayeux tapestry in France. That evening, the table became an altar when Father Paul spread a simple white cloth and arranged the chalice, the candle, the Bible and a plate holding a loaf of ordinary bread, especially baked for the occasion. The ordinary, the daily, combined in an extraordinary way with the mystical and the ancient as we listened to the words of Jesus the night before his death,

"This is my body, this is my blood - which will be given up for you."

As we shared the bread and wine in community, our sense of identity as "the body of Christ" expanded.

That night I lay awake for a long time, the people, images, feelings, lyrics resounding in my mind, a living portrait of the people of God.

LEAVE-TAKING

The night before Brian's transfer to Mount Vernon Hospital, Curt, I and the three younger children meet Father Paul in Brian's room for a brief prayer service. Father touches Brian with warmth and tenderness as he prays for him and for all of us. His words, "our failures and the times we've done what is right" somehow haunting. Curt says Brian had tears in his eyes when we left. I didn't see.

On December 12, we prepare for the move to Mount Vernon Hospital. Neil Henry helps pack up things in Brian's room– he will carry the stuffed dog with the sad face, a gift from Teresa. Janine, Brian's highly competent primary nurse, hugs him and tells us, "I've really learned a lot caring for Brian." The six-foot male nursing assistant grins, "I'll sure miss the parade of pretty girls who came to visit Brian." The Kaiser doctor of the week, yet another new face, comes in, shakes hands with my neighbor, saying, "How are you, Mrs.Rife."

A farewell note to the therapists:

> It's been painful for us who knew Brian before, to see him so diminished, and there were occasions when your lighthearted smiles and jokes seemed incongruent with what we were feeling. The good news is that it's a contagious attitude, and if we are coming to a better place in our emotions and our ability to relate to Brian as he is, you contributed to that change."

.3.

...INTO THE FIELDS OF LIGHT

–Euripides

MOUNT VERNON HOSPITAL

Brian lies on the stretcher as he is wheeled through the light-filled halls of Mount Vernon Hospital to his new room on 5A, the rehabilitation unit. It has been five months since Brian's accident plunged him into a long darkness. I walk beside him, carrying fading posters from hopeful friends, a paper bag full of T-shirts, and his high-top sneakers.

Since July the realization gradually dawned on all of us, family and friends, that Brian might never be the same person we knew before July 14, but in spite of that reality, there would be much to rejoice about as we watched him gradually increase in his capabilities. In the weeks ahead, sometimes we talked with the "old Brian"; sometimes he seemed an odd, even threatening stranger, and on days of grace and enlightenment, he became a charming, interesting, courageous survivor, worthy of our admiration and love.

In Brian's new room, the nurse on duty that day gives me a routine form to fill out. What does Brian eat, what time does he get up, go to sleep? Silly questions, I think to myself. Which Brian, the one who used to be? Is that Brian relevant any longer? I notice a box of Attends, adult paper diapers and the fact of Brian's inability to control such basic bodily functions registers anew in my conscious thinking.

While nurses and attendants set Brian up in his new room, taking his vital signs, changing the dressing on his trach, we walk into an adjoining recreation room where we meet a middle aged man in a wheelchair. His speech is labored, but we listen patiently and learn he is recovering from a stroke. He says he likes to read and is frustrated because of his double vision. We discuss getting the "talking books" from the library. My mind grasps some possible outcomes, visual difficulties, impaired speech, working my way to acceptance of whatever might be.

Finally we sit down on three plastic chairs outside Brian's room and speak with physiatrist Roger Gisolfi, a lean, intense, hard-working man, affectionately referred to by staff and patients as Dr. G. He is cautious, "Yes, we have seen some encouraging responses from Brian, but he is very fragile. He's got 45 things wrong with him medically, and every time you turn around something else goes wrong." He will make no predictions of success or failure, "Let's see where we are at the end of the 60 days Kaiser has agreed to fund."

Brian was immediately placed on a rigorous and well coordinated daily schedule. Speech therapy every morning with Judy Holmes; wet washcloths, bells, ice–sensory stimulation. Physical therapy twice a day with Mary Beth Ireland and assistants; bending and flexing Brian's knees, watching his balance in a sitting position. Primary nurses Chris Wade and Polly Martin bathed, fed and changed Brian, all the while keeping up constant conversation. Afternoon sessions with occupational therapist Adair Villareal, working with Brian to hold the washcloth and wipe his own face. Anyone who treated him repeated a similar message: "Brian, you were in a car accident. Now you're getting better. That's why I'm here. To help you move. To get your muscles to do things again."

Collectively, these young professionals were known as "the team" and met regularly to trade discoveries and map out ways to treat Brian. Their observations were faithfully recorded:

December 18 - team meeting

—Patient strengths: Inconsistent responses, demonstrating head righting in sitting, visual tracking with eye.

—Deficits: Rigid trunk, no vision in left eye.

—Nursing goals: Continue to turn and reposition every two hours. Suction trach one to two times each shift.

—Therapy Goals: Observe for responses to stimulation; develop yes/no responses.

We'd barely settled in to our new surroundings and begun to feel comfortable with the many faces of the team when we began to understand the next bureaucratic hurdle before us. Since Brian, a typical college student, had no assets of his own, we learned that he was eligible for Medicaid coverage for his rehabilitation when the 60 day Kaiser coverage ran out. BUT in order to secure coverage through the Virginia Medicaid system, he would have to be transferred to yet another hospital, probably in Richmond, two hours from our home, where we would have to get to know another new team of therapists! The current Medicaid rules allowed coverage only at certain approved hospitals.

WHAT CHILD IS THIS?

I am preparing a collage of pictures as a Christmas present for my parents. Danny and I find a 1965 photo, Honolulu airport. Pink flower leis resting on our shoulders, we are saying farewell to friends and our home for the past two and one half years. Curt holds two–year–old Scott in his arms and I carry Brian, in a reclining infantseat. Memories... Scott, energetic, curious and active; Brian, at five months, cuddly and pliable, smiling contentedly at every friendly face that looked his way. I tell Danny about the picture. He comments, "That's before Brian could drive a car."

When I visit Brian a week before Christmas dressed in my green suit, fresh from a luncheon with my book discussion group, dubbed the Ladies of the Club, I feel good about life and the hopefulness of our new surroundings. I reminisce with him about the gift he and Sheri gave me last Christmas, a copy of Ladies of the Club and how pleased I'd been with that gift.

A couple of days later I talk to Brian about Christmas, showing him pictures from a book, Images of God, vivid black and white drawings of the Hand of God (reminiscent of the Sistine chapel), Jacob Wrestling with an Angel, Jesus Raising Lazarus. I wonder about the quality of his eyesight. Does it matter? Does he see with his spirit? When I'm ready to leave, I ask him to give me a kiss good-bye. I kiss him on the cheek and hold my face close. He purses his lips, then parts them, emitting an audible smack. I don't allow myself to feel fully elated–too risky. I say, "Brian, that was great–I love you, I'll see you tomorrow."

Two days before Christmas, we have a photo session with Neil Henry and a Post photographer. Brian is reaching up to people, things, touching his face, his eyes, his ears, as though he is rediscovering himself.

The folk music group from our parish has arrived at the day room on 5B to sing Christmas carols for the fifth floor rehab patients. We've prearranged with recreational therapist Ellie Dailey to bring Brian and other interested patients into the day room for our singing. As we introduce ourselves, we wonder why Brian is not yet part of the group. Word comes that he can't leave his room because of a staph infection.

I feel defeated and find it difficult to keep a smile on my face as we sing, "Noel, noel," but somewhere behind the scenes, someone makes an exception. Brian is here now at the door, in the wheelchair, holding his head up with dignity. They wheel him in, oxygen and feeding tube hookup trailing behind. The atmosphere in the room changes, the singers take it all in and sing with renewed spirit, "What Child Is This."

I sense, too, more acceptance from the group we're singing for. Now we are part of them and the particular burdens they bear. From that point, I make eye contact with only Brian, feeling acceptance and love of him as he is now, without the crowding in of the pain of losing the Brian that was.

Christmas eve– hospital by 6:30, then carols, Mass and home for our traditional meal of beef fondue. We arrive at the hospital with a couple of presents for Brian: a memory game from Danny, a music tape from Sheri, a calendar from the Crandalls. We give Brian Danny's package and struggle through the process of opening it. How confused the stimuli sometimes are! He seems to want to participate but is unable to accomplish the task. I attempt to help his hands to do it, something I've seen therapists do. He looks at me with what seems to be anger and mouths expression that I take to mean, "No, don't do it for me!"

"You don't want me to do it. OK, Brian."

Scott's mind works on this challenge. "Come on, you're going to *work* on this," he says forcefully, but with an edge of uncertainty in his voice. Sheri is tender and expressive with Brian this evening. When the memory game is finally opened, Scott remembers that there's a similar game at home. Brian nods at him with understanding.

On Christmas day Curt, Karen and I visit Brian in the afternoon. I talk to him of the months since July –where he's been, what has happened, the help he is getting from the therapists. He is sitting in a chair holding his head up well. He is moving the left side of his mouth vigorously, attempting to speak. I tell him I wish I could understand and I'm glad he's trying.

When he is back in bed, he reaches out to me, and I say "Do you want to give me a hug?" Did I intuit or see an affirmative response? I don't know, but I place myself under his arm, my head on his chest. He reaches around me with the other arm and I feel pressure. He touches my hair. My eyes release warm tears onto his T-shirt. I feel the urge to weep with abandon but check the flow, believing it's OK for him to see a few tears but not a major flood!

I ask Curt and Karen on the way home, "Did he really touch my hair?" Could anyone else present sense what I sensed–Brian really in touch with me, Mom? "Yes," Karen says, "he was really responding." "Yes", Curt says, "he touched your hair."

Just after Christmas we meet again with Dr. Gisolfi. We suggest a rundown on Brian, top to bottom. Dr. G. demonstrates his awareness of each issue:

The eyes: "We're watching carefully, we'll not close the other eye without grave reasons; we don't want to cut out sensory input."

The jaw: "We're thinking it through, why he can't move it."

The feeding tube: "We want to feed him at intervals during the day and be able to unhook him for therapy sessions or other movement outside his room.

His legs, stiff and locked in a bent position: "The spasticity occurs for multiple reasons. We've decided not to give muscle relaxant shots; the therapists are doing OK with more conventional movement work."

NEW YEAR UPS...AND DOWNS

January 1

A visit to MVH followed by ice-skating at the Mount Vernon rink, a treat for Danny. We bring Brian's T-shirt from Fancy-Tee's with its mock tuxedo look. We show it to his nurse, Maggie, "How about this for New Year's!" She maneuvers him into the shirt, and we all find the effect very pleasing! I approach Brian and notice he is grimacing in a strange way. I comment, "I think something's coming up." It does. The day's feeding has not absorbed. Brown liquid on his tuxedo shirt. Maggie grabs a towel as more comes up.

Danny starts to look miserable, "When are we going skating?"

We go down to the cafeteria for coffee and let Brian rest. When we return, he is still upchucking. I feel exhausted and not much like ice-skating, more like going home to an aspirin. But we decide to keep our commitment to Danny. Before long, I've let go of Brian for the day and move around the ice beside Danny with abandon. In the evening we all go out to dinner. Somehow an animated discussion develops about Curt and me in our courtship days on the cabin cruiser exploring the Potomac.

Chatting, enjoying one another, enjoying our shrimp, crab legs, fries and cokes, prospects for 1986 seemed brighter.

INTO THE LIGHT

January 7, 1986

"Chris called from the hospital," Curt reports emphatically to me over the phone, "Brian spoke today! She put her finger over his trach and he said, 'Where am I?' and 'Why can't I talk?'" I want to feel joy, but my emotions are guarded, unwilling to board the rollercoaster again. I settle for the attitude, "I'll wait and see for myself."

Curt spends time with him during therapy that day and is brimming over with the experience of Brian's speaking. Curt had frequently prayed "Our Father, who art in Heaven..." with Brian when he ended his visits. Today, as he was leaving, he put his finger over the trach, and Brian joined in the prayer, "Give us this day our daily bread . . ." He told me later, "Then I knew there was a real being there, I would at least be able to hear his thoughts, even if they are scrambled." He calls his parents to tell them, then Scott. I am feeling left out because I've not yet heard the speaking for myself.

Danny and Eric come with me to the hospital that evening. We hover, trying to coax words out of him. He is very alert and his lips move, but we hear no sound as described by others. When we leave for home, though, some of the weight of the last six months lifts.

I arrive at 5A just as the physical therapy team is getting him into the chair. The first words I hear from him are, "I want to work." I am elated, *Brian lives* and he wants to *work* at restoring his life! But then he does not cooperate in the movement from bed to chair. Mary Beth's voice is soothing, her words slow and deliberate, "Brian, today is January 10 and we're your therapists here to work with you. You have a trach in your throat, you were in a car accident. Do you understand?"

"Yes... I unnerstan," Brian says, the words bursting forth uncertainly as the nurse holds a piece of gauze over the trach opening. Senses on edge, I lean closer.

Mary Beth goes on enthusiastically, "That was good. I understand you, too! We understand each other."

"Yes, that's nice," says Brian, as a warm ripple goes through the group looking on.

Then Brian says, "Sounds like I'm talking through..." The end of the sentence is unintelligible. When his nurse Chris joins us, she explains she'd said to him earlier, "Sounds like you're talking through your underwear!" He remembered a previous conversation, a very good sign!

"Do you have nickname?" Brian asks Mary Beth.

"Yes, it's Shump– my family calls me that. Do you have a nickname?"

"No," he replies. I mention Dingo, a name given him by dorm mates at Longwood, but it doesn't connect.

Suddenly, Brian becomes agitated, looking around him in confusion, "Animal, a dog . . ." Mary Beth picks up the floppy-eared dog on the windowsill, and places it near Brian's hand, asking him to touch it.

"Brian," she said slowly. "You're seeing things and you're not sure whether they're dreams or not. You've had a very bad injury to your brain. Because of the injury you can mix up what's real and what isn't real."

I come to the side of the bed, and Judy asks him to say "Hi, Mom." He doesn't, but he mouths with muted sound, "I love you." "I love you, Brian; you're a great guy," I respond.

By that evening, joy has taken me over, and I allow its fullness. "I feel like dancing!" I tell Curt. We call the Jenc's who took us camping in the Shenandoah in September and agree the night calls for a celebration. With an unmistakeable lightness in our movements and in our banter, we jitterbug, polka and slow-dance, finally dropping into bed after midnight, pleasantly exhausted.

One more fear can be laid to rest. Brian can communicate with us. Brian has shown all of us his will to live, and here at Mount Vernon Hospital, that will is being nourished and sustained. Now, more than ever, it seems unthinkable to move him to yet another hospital.

During the next few days, we begin to learn how Brian sees this new world of his, as he asserts himself in many ways. As Mary Beth attempts to help him into the wheelchair, he says, "I don't need a wheelchair!" totally unaware of the actual limitations of his body. Once in the chair, he wants to leave the room. The team goes with his cues. Mary Beth helps him move his feet on the floor in a stepping motion. He becomes fixated on entering the nurse's station. That afternoon we observe two physical therapists who have not previously worked with Brian encouraging him to sit up on the side of the bed. He makes a fist and says clearly, "Get out of here!" When I speak with my father on the phone, relating this incident, he is pleased, "He's still got some fight in him then!"

Another day, I take him for a ride in the wheelchair. When we stop to

look out the window, he says, "Where's my ride?" so we get right on it. We
meet the mother of another patient and I introduce him. He says hello,
shakes her hand, then says, "I keep spilling my beer." He is off in another
time and place. We take the elevator to the first floor and tour the bright,
spacious therapy room, commenting on the equipment, the mirror, the huge
rubber ball. Back upstairs, Brian looks at some of his fellow patients, "Who
are all these people? They look retarded." He has no awareness that he looks
much like the others.

On the 14th of January, we meet with the team. Dr. G's overview:
"We have a whole new chapter now. The question a month ago was, would
Brian wake up. Now he has. Three areas we will be concerned with:

— his ability to move various parts of his body in appropriate ways.
  Not all movement is good movement–an oversimplified rule of
  thumb, if it looks normal, it's probably good;
— cognition, his ability to comprehend, learn, think; and
— behavior, processing of multiple stimuli, difficult for him at this point.

Two things tend to happen with over-stimulation, shut down or
agitation. A well-trained visitor will know how to read these signs."

A few days later, as I talk with him, Brian blows air out the side
of his mouth, sort of a "poof, poof." I laugh, partly joy at seeing him do
anything, even the most minimal, bizarre anythings and partly because
it is funny! But he chastises me, "It's not funny!" I apologize. Later I
spend long moments just looking at him, trying to read him, then I read
to him from one of his Louis L'Amour paperbacks.

THE COUNTDOWN

We now have less than 30 days left of Kaiser funding. Brian has
dramatically shown his determination to live and work at the essence of
life. Neil Henry has heard Brian speaking. Surely now he has enough
material to finish his story; surely the system can change and allow us
to keep Brian where he is making progress.

Betsy Zeigler, the social worker has spoken with Pat Davis at
Kaiser-Permanente to request continued funding for Brian–no leeway.
We consider our next step. Dr. G. will write to Kaiser, describing
Brian's progress and expressing his belief that a move would be
detrimental to his rehabilitation.

Our congressional representative suggests we write to James

Kenley, a commissioner with the State Department of Health in Richmond. We receive a "bureaucratic" answer. Mount Vernon Hospital has been evaluated for approval as a Medicaid facility, but the process for this approval will take from 3 to 6 months. There must be a public hearing, then comments back to the board, and finally the Governor has 30 days to review the case.

I start thinking "like a lawyer." I remember that Claire Guthrie, formerly an attorney with Hogan and Hartson, has taken a position in Richmond in the new Baliles administration. I call her office and tell her secretary I am sending some material describing our situation. Twenty days to go.

Finally, on February 1st, I receive a memo from Claire Guthrie in Richmond. Having consulted with an Assistant Attorney General, she writes:

> *A resolution is not anticipated prior to the end of 1986. Two problems arise; the first involves the fact that Mt. Vernon Hospital is a Medicaid approved "acute-care hospital" (short-term), rather than a "long-term care facility." As such, MVH is subject to the Medicaid regulation limiting payment for hospitalization to a period not in excess of twenty one days. The conflict arising out of the application of the "21 day rule" is in the process of being resolved and there lies the second problem. Six Medicaid directors toured Mt. Vernon's facility in early '85 and were convinced of the need for a change in policy. Unfortunately, such a change cannot be accomplished without following the Administrative Process Act (APA). Even under an accelerated scenario, this matter is unlikely to be resolved prior to September or October of 1986.*

Then at the bottom of the page, a footnote pointing us in the right direction.

> *The Code of Virginia excludes the following from the APA process:*
>
> *"Regulations which an agency finds are necessitated by an emergency situation. In such cases the agency shall state in writing the nature of the emergency and of the necessity for such action and may adopt such regulations with the prior approval of the Governor."*

Claire's memo points out that the Governor defines what is an "emergency" and if the emergency regulation is approved, it is approved for the limited time it takes to complete the APA process. Claire also gives me the address of a lawyer in Alexandria who has "political clout." Sounds good, so I send him a full copy of material sent to Governor Baliles. At the advice of a neighbor, I also write our state senator, Joseph Gartlan.

We have nine days left of funding.

Friends and neighbors have already agreed to write letters in our behalf. Now we revise our request for letters directly to Governor Baliles instead of the commissioners at the State Department of Health. As one friend, a 50's West Point graduate, pointed out, "You're writing to a bunch of Lieutenant, colonels. You need to get to the general." Approximately 15 articulate letters are on their way to Richmond. Eric's 8th grade English teacher guides her class in writing to Baliles. Hospital personnel write; one of the most touching letters is sent by Chris, Brian's primary nurse:

Dear Governor Baliles:

Rehabilitation of a brain injured patient takes a lot of courage, a lot of love, a lot of time and patience, a lot of trust, and a lot of consistency.

It is a traumatic experience waking up from a coma, not knowing where you are, what has happened to you, why you cannot remember the people standing in front of you, and why other people have to meet your every need...

Each day I see more and more of Brian emerge as he assists with bathing and dressing and his sense of humor returns. A move at this time will hinder the remarkable progress Brian has made and cause him to regress. The trust that took so long to build will be destroyed and Brian will have to learn new faces and behaviors, and try to trust new people.

Please help the Rifes.

On my trips back and forth to the hospital, the blue LTD Ford station wagon has become my cocoon as I make the 30 minute drive, usually during the day, Curt and the children visiting in the evenings. The music of country western singer Dan Seals feeds my spirit:

My father said, some things you learn,
by only doin' when it comes your turn,
Everything comes around, so be ready if you can,
Prepare your heart, like the farmer turns the land.

You plant your fields when the spring is tender,
When the summer beats down, you pray for rain,
You hope for the harvest, the long cold winter,
Then you plant your fields again... plant your fields again.
                                    —*Seals (See references)*

BREAKTHROUGH

We wait. Tension builds in the family. I fight with Curt about socks in the laundry room, with Eric about spilled milk and dishes not put away. I'm angry with Neil, because there is no chance of the <u>Post</u> story coming out in time to be of help. On the 6th of February, I wake up with murderous plotting on my mind. I will refuse to sign the papers to have him moved! I will go to a TV news program. God, I don't want to lose this battle! What are my deepest motivations at this point, helping Brian or beating the system? Moments of anger at Brian too– the incredible repercussions of a night of beer-drinking and an impulsive decision to drive to the beach. I pray for some serenity in the midst of it all, and it comes, almost against my will!

Phone call from Kaiser-Permanente. In spite of Dr. G's letter explaining Brian's progress, they are firm in their decision to fund only through the 12th of February. A letter arrives from Ray Sorrell, the Director of Virginia Medical Assistance Services, apparently the man responsible for coordinating the change in the Medicaid system. Mr. Sorrell relates that his son died of muscular dystrophy, and he is genuinely sensitive to our situation but says nothing can be done to expedite the approval.

With only a week of funding left, we consider how we might survive a move to Richmond. Friends whose parents live in Richmond suggest I could stay with them for a few weeks while getting Brian settled in Sheltering Arms Hospital. But I haven't given up.

On February 9th, with three days left, I attend a bridal shower, fighting my misery. From another guest, I pick up one more lead, a state representative in Alexandria. I tell Danny it's like being in the last five minutes of a soccer game and being down 4 to 1. I've got to try to kick a few more goals; the odds are against it, but I'll track down this last lead. I am unable to reach him the next day.

On February 11th, State Senator Gartlan calls me to say he met Claire Guthrie over the weekend at a social gathering and they discussed

Brian's case. He feels it is important enough to take the situation to the governor. I'm elated! He asks me to have Dr. G. write a letter describing the detrimental effects a move would have on Brian at this point in his recovery. He asks if there is anyone else who would be affected by the changed rules. I find out there is another boy at Fairfax Hospital who could be transferred to MVH if it were Medicaid approved. In the evening I call Senator Gartlan to give him this information. He sounds less certain, "I don't want to get your hopes up." I sit at the typewriter and write three pages of what I'd say to the governor if I had just 20 minutes of his time.

February 12

I work at Hogan and Hartson, ragged and unwilling to function at the typewriter. Just before I leave for home, Curt calls: "Just talked to Dr. G.; they've been conferring with Richmond. Negotiations are coming along just fine and Mount Vernon has decided to keep Brian as a 'guest' for six weeks until negotiations are complete." My mind has considerable trouble processing this latest miracle. I wait till I'm home to hear it again. A meeting took place in the Governor's office; they decided the process could be shortened after all. Approval can be in place by the first of April. Mount Vernon administration decided they could absorb the costs under these special circumstances. Incredible; ranks right up there with the parting of the Red Sea! Who did what; what happened? We don't know. Curt says, "Just thank everybody," and we do. Flowers to the fifth floor at the hospital, a call to Senator Gartlan, who says, "I wish I could take credit for the breakthrough, but I didn't have a chance to talk to him."

After a week of recouping energies and settling down to our new realities, I experience a real psychological and spiritual letdown. This battle is won. Like my hero Don Quixote, I have been jousting windmills, beating unbeatable foes. Now we must face our needs and Brian's condition and decide how we can work with the rehab staff to bring Brian as far as possible.

.4.

THE RACE IS NOT TO THE SWIFT...

–Ecclesiastes

No one could predict how long Brian's rehabilitation would take, but we knew already from other families that the journey would be long and tedious. We were told that periods of progress were often followed by discouraging plateaus. We were less aware that progress and plateaus would also describe the adjustments required in our family. The National Head Injury Foundation logo reads: "Because life after head injury may never be the same." True for the survivor and equally so for his family; each member of that family, parents and siblings, adjusts to this truth in a unique way. The family system, too, is forever altered.

Trips to the hospital –a 30 minute drive each way– became part of our routine four or five times a week. Regular meetings with the team and Dr. G. were scheduled, where we shared encouragement, frustrations and progress. Writing of this period, nearly five years later, I am filled with melancholy, wondering why I can't remember much about interactions with our other children. Scott was in his junior year at Virginia Tech, Sheri was a senior in high school, Eric in 8th grade and Danny in 4th grade. Although I know we tried to be aware, our time with them had to be inadequate. Brian's needs always seemed compelling.

Somewhere in the many sessions we'd had with specialists since July, someone had indicated, "Most recovery occurs within the first year." Setting a time limit on expectations is widely discredited among rehabilitation professionals now, but for us in the early part of 1986, this thought created tension between our expectations and the patience advised by the rehabilitation team at Mount Vernon Hospital. For better or worse, the process of Brian's rehabilitation shaped our lives.

Many parts of Brian's brain were still not awake and functioning, even though he now could speak and react to his surroundings in some fundamental ways. One writer describes the dilemma of the traumatically injured brain this way:

> [The injured person] has fallen through a gap in medical knowledge much the way Alice slipped down a hole into Wonderland. The brain –how it thinks, creates, remembers– is still mostly a mystery. It is a world where science collides with philosophy and religion, producing a paradox of which Lewis Carroll would be proud; a brain that cannot completely comprehend itself. (*Elliot, see references*)

However incomplete a nuts and bolts approach may be to the healing of a human mind, Mount Vernon's therapy program was the best available. Under the guidance of Dr. Gisolfi, therapists and nurses divided up the many physical and cognitive challenges of Brian's rehabilitation and went to work.

Movement

The first physical challenges to be met were unlocking Brian's jaw and helping him achieve some control of his leg and trunk movements. His body lay in the bed as if paralyzed, but he had no spinal cord injury. Since the long period in coma, his jaw had become frozen in place, even though the wiring had been removed before he was released from shock trauma in Baltimore. Eating and improved communication skills depended on his ability to move his lower jaw. An early report on Brian indicated his mouth opening was only half a centimeter, "due to reflex bite plus mandibular fractures and soft tissue contracture." Dr. Fiorucci, an oral surgeon, performed "manipulation of the mandible" under anesthesia in mid-March. After this procedure, speech therapist Judy Holmes worked with him daily, till August 11th, when she recorded in the communication book we kept by his bed that he had achieved mouth opening of 2.9 centimeters!

Judy's unsophisticated tools were tongue depressors wrapped with surgical tape in groups of graduated sizes. Six blades stacked together measured 1 centimeter, eight measured 1.2 centimeters and so on. Each day the first order of business during Judy's session with Brian would be to start with the smallest stack, gently but firmly positioning it between his teeth, then in 10 minutes trying the next size up.

Because eating and communicating skills ranked high in my hopes for Brian, I sat in on many of Judy's sessions with him. I will never forget the seeming incongruity of placing a stack of wooden sticks in his mouth and then asking him to speak. Reminded me of Eliza Doolittle in "My

Fair Lady" trying to say "The rain in Spain falls mainly in the plain" with her mouth full of marbles! Brian became somewhat fixated on the sticks and would put them in his mouth at other times. We would walk in and find him sitting there with this huge "dragon tooth" protruding from his mouth.

One day I sat in on therapy and heard the following conversation with Judy's fingers in Brian's mouth:

Brian: "Not again!"

Judy: "I'm afraid so."

Brian: "I'm going to bite it off."

Judy: "You wouldn't do that."

Brian: "Probably not."

Judy's entries in the communication book we kept by his bed illustrate his slow but sure progress in jaw opening and eating. Other strategies included a lollipop and the suggestion that we could help by trying to get him to yawn or open his mouth as frequently as possible.

During the last week of March, Brian began to recognize the nature of this relationship. "You called me your teacher today and recalled my name twice during our session," read Judy's entry one day. In April and May, Judy's goals for her sessions with Brian expanded to include dry swallowing, then liquids and food, the first "real" food he had consumed in nine months! On one early try, he had six sips of orange drink, but was unable to swallow and the liquid had to be suctioned back out. By the end of May, his swallow reflex had become more reliable, and he was able to consume ice cream, pudding and baby foods.

Looking at his first meal of gravy, mashed potatoes, jello, milk and green soup, he said, "It may not be as good as I thought!" I was there that day to help if needed. It was like a trip back in time to the infant Brian's first meals in the high chair. Getting the spoon to his mouth took all his energy, so I offered to help, which proved to be a tricky proposition. He finally asked me to leave when we reached a certain level of mutual frustration, and I did.

In those first five months of 1986, during the same period when he was opening his mouth and learning to eat, physical therapists Mary Beth Ireland and Buffi Smith worked with Brian daily to improve his leg and trunk control. Their sessions involved trips to the mat room, where, with infinite patience, they placed him in different positions, standing, sitting, kneeling, or moving his legs to gradually reduce the stiffness. They too recorded progress in the communication book. At the end of March,

> *"We worked with you in bed, curling you up like a ball and rocking and rolling. You worked hard and allowed us to do a lot of tough things. You held your head up without support and used your feet to propel the wheelchair."*

But other days, Brian was unaware, "Brian, we could not awaken you for anything!" or unwilling, "You said you wanted to go home so you could sleep, but I told you your mom wouldn't let you sleep either!" By the beginning of May, Brian could transfer himself from bed to wheelchair with minimum assistance, and by the middle of June, physical therapists wrote: "You are getting better control of your body. Hang in there, you are getting well!" By early July, they worked on standing and began the early stages of walking. At the end of July, we watched him walking with Mary Beth's expert guidance, "I want to do it, I will do it!" he said. By this time Brian was back to his pre-accident weight, 147 pounds.

As Brian gained more control of his body, the risk of his falling became greater. His judgment about what he could do and what he could not do was often inaccurate, a typical situation with survivors of traumatic brain injury. One entry in the book reflects efforts to improve Brian's judgment of his limits: "You agreed to try and trust people when they tell you things. I'm worried about your safety. It's hard to be patient, but try so you don't get injured."

During this period, the staff suggested a "playpen" arrangement in Brian's room. A plywood structure, about 6 feet by 6 feet was constructed in the center of the room, with mattresses on the floor. Short of having someone with him at all times, it seemed the only way to assure his safety. That arrangement was never acceptable to him, however, and was dismantled in a couple weeks. The next idea was a system of tiered mattresses, with the bed against the wall, two mattresses beside it and one beside that. This way it was almost impossible for him to hurt himself getting out of bed. He found it handy in other ways too, telling a neighbor one day that his bed was wet that night, but "no problem, I just rolled down to the next bed!"

The other precaution Dr. G. insisted upon for his safety was a helmet. They suggested a biker's helmet, which we promptly purchased, but he refused to keep it on his head. Then we remembered a batter's helmet at home and brought it in. That coincided with Brian's pre-accident image of himself, little league baseball star, and he agreed to wear it.

I remember this period as one of high stress for us. At one point Brian tipped over the wheelchair and had a huge bump on his head. We felt frustrated with the staff at Mount Vernon at that point, but in retrospect, they were doing all they could do to assure his safety, short of using restraints to keep him in the bed, which would surely have been damaging to him psychologically. It's easy to imagine how this mobile, yet unaware, stage could be mishandled by people less knowledgeable about the tedious process of recovery.

Along with directing his progress in eating and mobility, Brian's two primary nurses, Chris Wade and Polly Martin, were responsible for Brian's basic physical care and helping him to re-learn the activities of daily living, known as ADL's in rehab lingo. They assisted him with toilet training, dressing, toothbrushing, showering. Their notes in the book were earthy and humorous. Sometimes they had his cooperation and sometimes not. "Today while I was changing Brian, he told me to 'shut up, I'm in a violent mood tonight.' I told him he needed to control his anger and that I was there to help him." A few days later, "Brian was very cooperative with his care. At first he didn't want me to wash his hair because he couldn't pay me, but when I started, he said, 'You can do this all day if you want to!'"

The first week of May, the trach tube, inserted in Brian's neck to keep him breathing when he entered the University of Maryland shock-trauma unit, finally came out. No stitches were used to close the opening; it healed itself in a few days. Brian would wear the "badge" of his ordeal in that telling indentation. Polly wrote, "Hey, Brian–great news! The doctor pulled out your trach tube today. You're relaxed now and breathing comfortably."

Toilet training and personal care skills moved along slowly but surely. By early June, "You used the urinal 2 out of 3 times tonight," and "You brushed your own teeth at the sink, rinsing your mouth three times. Keep up the good work." The ability to shower by himself was gradually regained, but not before some soapsuds and waterspray free-for-alls. I came in one day to help Chris with this process. Brian's frustration boiled over, and he called us "incompetent women." I decided to skip the showers!

After those many months when Brian was fed only through the tube, we were all thrilled to see him eat normally again. Chris wrote: "What a typical guy you turned out to be, ate everything in sight, then asked for more! I told you that you would get fat and you laughed and said, 'Who gives a shit. I'm making up for lost time.'"

The extraordinary degree of Chris's personal and professional commitment to Brian are evident in this entry in the book, one of the last made:

> *You fell out of the chair after lunch, but you were OK. You punched me once and you were irked at me. I gave you a pillow and you said, "I can't believe it. I was so mean to you and you gave me a pillow to make me comfortable." Before I left, you kissed my hand and asked me to say prayers with you. We said the "Our Father." No matter what happens, Brian, I won't stop being your nurse, whether you are mad at me or not.*

Cognition

Cognition is defined as the process of knowing in the broadest sense, including perception, memory, and judgment. During the first half of 1986, the state of Brian's "knowing" was elusive and complex. The intricate mental processes of recognition, memory and comprehension were drastically altered, and we could always expect the unexpected in our relationship with him. To further complicate matters, his vision and hearing were impaired, but till late summer his responses were not reliable enough to evaluate these senses accurately. Once, in those early months, I remember standing by his bed saying, "Brian, it's me, Mom!" He looked at me quizzically, "You sure as hell don't look like Mom!" Was it a deficit in his vision, his memory, his retrieval system, or the processing of information from sensory to speech? Perhaps all of the above. No one really knows.

Sometimes he recognized people, but used a name different from the one he would normally have used. For example, before my parents came for a visit in March, I tried to prepare him by showing him pictures. "Do you see your grandma and grandpap (the names he always used for them)?" He studied the picture, "Who are these people?" Then, "It is my grandfather and grandmother." On the day they visited, he reacted to them knowingly, but the names were a bit off, "It's my *god*father" and "Hi, Grandmother." When Curt's mother visited, he called out, "It's Eva Mae!" instead of Grandmother Rife, his usual way of addressing her. Similarly, he would see an object and recognize some of its characteristics but not know how to integrate the information. One day in the spring during a walk outdoors, I picked a hyacinth from the flower bed and invited Brian to smell it; he attempted to eat it instead!

As erratic as his mental processes were, he was frequently able to come out with a quick-witted response to a situation. One day when my parents visited, Judy Holmes arrived for her session with him. "Hi, Brian," she greeted him, "I'm your speech therapist." He shot back, "Shit, everybody's my speech therapist!" Like the story of the hand-squeeze in shock-trauma, my father loved this one and used it for weeks when people inquired about Brian. Later in the year, my sister brought him a package which contained a red Adidas tee shirt. He opened it, grinned and said, "You know what that stands for, All Day I Dream About Sex." That, too, became the anecdote of the week.

But the younger generation found it more difficult to relate to Brian's arduous progress. Sheri, Eric and Danny visited Brian rarely, and I wondered how they could adjust to the new Brian if they didn't spend more time with him. Once in April, Sheri came with me and asked him tentatively, "Do you know who I am?" He replied, "I knew you the first time I saw you. Your name is Sheri; you didn't think I knew it." Although this was an encouraging visit for her, she still found it difficult and painful to relate to him.

I discussed my concerns about Brian's at-home siblings with the social worker. She suggested that we plan a picnic on the grassy areas on the hospital grounds; just being outside might help. "So often," she said, "children find the atmosphere of the hospital oppressive." It seemed like good advice, so in the afternoon on Mother's Day we brought a picnic lunch, some blankets, the dog, pudding and Coke for Brian. The younger boys *were* more comfortable, talking to Brian and playing a little catch with him. For those few hours, we concentrated on the logistics of a picnic lunch –helping Brian with his pudding, keeping the napkins from blowing away, sharing munchies– shifting the focus from Brian. If his participation was limited from our point of view, for him it was a pleasantly exhausting outing in the sun and fresh spring air.

At this time, because Brian was making significant progress on all fronts, the limitations of the hospital environment frustrated him. He began asking about when he could come home. Over the next months, this became a contentious subject. Most of the time, he did not accept the facts that were being repeated to him daily by therapists, nurses, family. "Brian, you were in a car accident; this is Mount Vernon Hospital; you've been here for six months." His short term memory was functioning only in fragmented ways. Because the events of recent weeks and months were not being recorded in his mind, he found it very hard to believe the stories of others.

He began to develop a conspiracy theory about the hospital. We were all making up this wild story to keep him trapped there. Curt wrote in the book the first of June, "You were unhappy with me for telling you about the accident. You wanted to go home and asked why I was leaving you here. I told you people here knew how to care for you."

Neuropsychologist Dr. Peter Patrick, began working with Brian in groups and individually during this period. He described Brian's behavior this way, "He does not shrink from physical challenges [he was working well with therapists], but resists informational challenges." He advised, "Smooth on by them for now."

With me, Brian's resistance took a particularly hostile form. During my visits in July, he confronted me repeatedly, "What is this all about? Why are you keeping me here. I'm 21, I want to be in college." I tried to stay with these conversations, dealing with the various questions as directly and calmly as possible. He let me know when I was raising my voice and I let him know the same. Much as I tried to remain objective, these words coming from him hurt me deeply. If he couldn't grasp even the minimal facts about his condition, how could he begin to understand how hard I'd fought for his life since July 14? One day he shouted at me to "Get out!" I stopped visiting for several weeks to protect myself from these hurtful exchanges and to allow him time to move beyond this stage.

During that time, he called home on the phone, saying, "Why am I here–you'll be lucky if I stay here!" Then he said something I didn't understand and I told him so. He replied, "Read my lips!" I told him, "I love you," and hung up, wishing some more positive thoughts could be programmed into his fractured thinking. He asked one friend who visited if he could come live with her when he got better if his family didn't want him.

Curt had a good instinct about the value of repeating positive ideas in his conversations with Brian. Curt would usually take him down to the cafeteria for a root beer during his evening visits. He wrote this note in July,

> "I have been telling you for the past few months that you are a winner. Tonight I asked what you were and you said, 'I am a winner and I make things happen, and I am going to get well.' You are getting much better, understanding and remembering more."

We wondered if more contact with the outside world might help him integrate all this information better. The artificial environment of the hospital sometimes keeps people with brain injury from grasping and dealing with their realities. Although many rehab programs now incorporate this fact into the therapeutic process, the consensus of

Brian's rehab team was against a home visit so soon. They believed the possible behavioral problems that might result from a visit home outweighed the possible benefits. So we did not press the issue.

The way outside contact can help was evident as we walked Brian around the hospital grounds in the wheelchair during the hospital's spring festival in mid-May. His brother Scott, who had joined the rescue squad at Virginia Tech, explained some of the rescue equipment on display (an ambulance and a helicopter) and gradually engaged Brian in discussion about all that had happened to him. "I was in an accident," Brian repeated slowly, "They came for me in an ambulance... then I was in a helicopter."

Gradually as spring moved into summer, his realities became clearer to him. The meaning of another mother's comment became clearer to me, "The better he gets, the worse he'll feel."

As his mind cleared enough to comprehend how poorly his body was working, he began to grieve his losses. The coordinated, athletic body that once moved according to his commands was gone. Polly recorded this in July,

> "You continue to impress everyone with how much better you're getting, alertness, orientation and vocabulary. But it also is a very difficult time for you. Realizing and accepting some of the problems is frustrating. You said, 'I can't believe I've missed a year of my life,' and later, 'I can't believe I'm such a cripple.' I told you that was not so and that you were doing great. *Keep Thinking Positive!*"

Occupational therapists began about this time to plan more complex tasks for Brian as his mental acuity improved. Rosemary Fleury continued the process of improved ADL's and began to incorporate writing and interpretation tasks, often using the computer. In June she wrote, "Brian scored 100% when asked to identify one picture/number/letter that was different from the other three on the screen," and "Brian put on his left shoe but needed assist with right shoe." Occupational therapists also assessed how well Brian could interpret bodily sensations and movement, "Brian could not distinguish hot from cold but he did accurately describe what his legs felt like–tight, loose, out more, in more–during therapy."

In July, evaluation of Brian's vision began. When asked to look at an eye chart, he said, "I can only see a white square on the door." Gradually it was determined that he could read large letters effectively with his left eye, but that vision in his right eye was severely limited. During his work in occupational therapy, he continued to integrate information about his actual limitations. "I feel so clumsy," when playing cards, and "I used to be able to just put on my socks without even looking; now it's a task!" But with patient repetition and work, steady improvement occurred. By November Rosemary wrote that Brian "can now use entire keyboard on computer using his new glasses." The glasses merely magnified. He typically challenged himself to do better on the computer, paddle ball game and bean bag throws. One day my parents and I watched his therapy session, and he said, "I like the audience, sort of a cheering section."

FIFTEEN MINUTES OF FAME

As Neil Henry of The Washington Post journeyed with us through Brian's awakening at Mount Vernon Hospital, he began to envision our story as a four–part series in the newspaper. The front page articles began on June 8th, 1986, entitled "Patient No. 18,874." For a few weeks, we experienced the intensity of the public eye, reminding us of Andy Warhol's statement, "In the future, everyone will be world famous for fifteen minutes."

We received dozens of letters and cards in response to the series. Many contained religious messages, "Pray to Jesus, the great physician;" "Our prayers are with you." Many others, including a District of Columbia police and fire department chaplain, applauded our "courage" and our "willingness to tell our story in such a full and revealing way." From a D.C. woman, " I lost my 21 year old son in a car accident. I was never given a chance to make any decision about his medical treatment as he died before reaching the hospital. So many people have told me I was fortunate he did not live to be a 'vegetable.'[5] I would have given anything to have kept him alive in any way possible. There is nothing I can ever do to help my son again."

And from a high school classmate of Curt's, who pondered "the luck of surviving to adulthood at all, considering all of the dumb things we did back then; we rode with incompetents and show-offs. . . . Somehow we made it through high school, taking chances and being lucky that we weren't maimed or into big trouble."

5. Richard Linn (RRTC, NY), proposes that "the term 'vegetable' never be used to refer to a human being." A legitimate medical term is "vegetative state."

We received many phone calls, expressing similar sentiments, but one was different. A man called and spoke with me at great length. A Roman Catholic father of eight, he related to me, his voice breaking, that reading the series had brought him to tears, as he remembered his daughter's accident seven years earlier. He said, "At the time, I couldn't cry; I had to be the tough Irishman."

His daughter was alive, but severely disabled. This man had kept his grief submerged all those years and was finally able to let it out as he read of our experience.

Mount Vernon Hospital had the series reprinted in booklet form to give to families when their sons, daughters and spouses came to the rehabilitation unit. Every few months, in the ensuing years, we have heard from someone who says, "We read your story; it gave us hope when we had none."

THE FAMILY

One of Dr. Peter Patrick's favorite themes when addressing family members is the fact that families so often burn themselves out while the brain injury survivor in the family is hospitalized, feeling that they have to be present daily and participate in every decision. They realize belatedly that they ought to be storing up energy for the day when the patient re-enters the home scene. "While he's in the hospital, he's got a whole crew of people looking after him. Stay home more often and take care of your own needs," he would repeat to families.

In the late summer of 1986, that advice took a firmer hold in our minds. As Brian continued to progress on all fronts, some of our anxieties were eased. We could begin to envision the process of bringing him home by the end of the year and feel assured that his ability to take care of himself was improving slowly but surely. As we stayed away from the hospital during that time to avoid the "when can I come home" battles, we saw the wisdom of taking a long vacation with the younger boys. For years, we had planned to take a trip west to visit friends in South Dakota and Montana. We discussed with the rehabilitation staff the possibility of taking this trip, and they agreed that it was a "healthy" plan for us to get away for a while. Certainly our level of trust in the Mount Vernon Hospital staff was total. The idea crystallized into an itinerary, and by August, we were on a plane headed for Rapid City, South Dakota with Eric and Danny. We sent postcards and notes printed in large letters to Brian from each stop in South Dakota and Montana.

With Brian in the background, Curt and I saw more clearly during our 18-day vacation the gaps in our relationship with Eric, now ready to enter high school, and Danny, ready for 5th grade. Deluded mom and dad that we were, we imagined these two young sons would be so delighted to have some "quality" time with their beleaguered parents, they would behave with perfect decorum and gratitude. Not so. After ten minutes at Mount Rushmore, "OK, we've seen it, now let's go." At dinner with Don Resset, who had written us the year before and was now our host in Montana, Eric commented, "Is this what we're having–it doesn't look very good." Don, a widower, and fortunately a long-time and understanding friend, had worked hard cooking and ministering to us, well aware of the challenges we'd faced in the past year. As a music teacher in the local intermediate school, he recognized the boys' behavior was a bit more chaotic than average and suggested gently their need for attention and occasional correction. Perhaps we should have recognized some of the underlying issues, but we did not. We just dealt with the behavior as well as we were able and trusted our friends for acceptance and forgiveness.

We returned at the end of August, and the boys began school. It was time to focus on home and to think through the impact on the family of Brian's return home. As our focus shifted to home, our visits to the hospital were limited to once or twice a week during the fall months.

● ● ●

During a visit with Brian the first of September, he and I went out to the deck where we had a congenial discussion about how long he'd been in the hospital and the possibility of a home visit soon. He agreed to visit the chapel with me, a quiet triangular shaped room near the center of the first floor of Mt. Vernon Hospital. When we were inside, Brian insisted on getting out of the chair and sitting on one of the cushioned benches with me. I felt a moment of panic, not certain I could handle this transfer alone. Brian's weight had increased to 155 pounds now and I'd always had a backup person on hand before. I decided that God would not let him fall here—not necessarily in line with my overall theology about what God does and does not do—but the thought calmed me as I helped him to the bench with only a little lurching. "May I sing a song," I asked him. He didn't hear and understand me at first. He yelled, "What?" "Do you mind if I sing a song," I yelled back. He said OK. I sang, "Be not afraid/ I go before you always/ come follow me/ and I will give you rest..." He sat back and relaxed, and when I was finished, he sighed, "That was nice." One of the "high places."

The first week of September, we finally had arranged for Brian's first visit home since the accident. We were more than a little anxious about how this visit would go and had been talking about it for several days. He called us on the phone Friday night, quite unaware of the implications for his family of this event, "I wanted to make sure you got the message to pick me up on Sunday." Right, Brian.

We decide to keep this visit very simple. No meal, just some sherbet and maybe mashed peaches. No visitors, just sitting on the patio for a while, allowing him to take the conversation anywhere he chose. Dr. Patrick had mentioned the possibility of "emotional flooding" and cautioned that when he was tired, we could expect some regression. At 1:15 we had him in the car, moving towards Springfield. In the front seat with Curt, looking at the suburban landscape, he commented, "Everything looks blurry." We realized this was the first time he had experienced his impaired vision from the inside of a car. When we arrived at the house, we gingerly managed the wheelchair up the two front steps and in the front door. Inside Eric and Danny showed him the computer, purchased since he was home. They invited him to play one of the games, but he quickly realized how slow his reactions were compared to his younger brothers and he wheeled away. Sitting on the patio, we shared a snack, and he discussed his physical problems–his jaw, his eyes–very lucidly.

By 4:15 when we came back inside, he seemed regressed and began the "I want to know why I'm in the hospital" questioning. I disengaged quickly and remembered the warning about fatigue. Before he left, we all gathered in a circle to say a prayer of thanks for the day, asking for continued healing and courage for Brian and for us. We drove him back to Mount Vernon at 5:00. We were all emotionally spent.

Brian's eventual return home, still months away, would be a big issue for all of us. This brief first visit provided a small glimpse into the process of re-integrating him into home and family. We had come a long way from the days when he was in a coma and unable to respond to us in any way. Still, we had a long way to go.

The third week in September we met with the rehabilitation team. I described it in my journal as "the all-time upbeat hospital meeting in fifteen months!" Dr. G. said, "Brian continues to exceed our expectations in all areas, memory, cognitive and physical." Each member of the team, physical, speech, and occupational therapies and nursing gave a glowing report of Brian's progress. Still there were additional issues to be resolved. Brian was unable to chew solid food, so he was to have an appointment with an oral surgeon to evaluate him for surgery to reposition his lower jaw. Somehow during the long process of mouth opening, it had become mis-aligned. Orthodontic work was also suggested to help in correcting his bite. Therapists had become more certain that Brian had severe hearing loss; an audiologist would evaluate him within the next week. All things considered, the therapy team rated Brian's outcome to be excellent.

TRANSITIONS

But from the point of view of home, the emotional, social and logistical issues surrounding Brian's return were only beginning to be considered. Brian was a totally different person from the carefree young man who left for the beach one night sixteen months ago. For his siblings, especially Eric, he must have seemed like a stranger. Even though there had been signals during our trip west, we were quite unaware of the extent of Eric's distress.

One day in October, Eric said he did not want to go to school. As we talked, I realized he was hurting deeply and knew he needed professional help.

After several sessions with a psychiatrist, we learned that Eric was grappling with some very difficult questions, in addition to the ordinary stresses of being fourteen. What was the point, he wondered, in studying math and English and social studies, when a person's life could be so drastically altered in an instant, as he had seen happen to his once handsome, vitally alive brother? Dr. Stein suggested that family counseling would be the best approach, an opportunity for all of us to air our painful emotions and fears during this time of transition as we prepared for Brian's return home.

Although we think our family has many strengths, we are not very adept at talking openly about feelings, a trait shared by many families. For myself, throughout the period since Brian's accident, I had recorded thoughts and feelings in my journal and in that way dealt with many fears, hopes, and angers. A journal entry on Brian's 21st birthday in April, for instance, noted one of my "rules" of survival, "Feel what you are feeling, as it comes to you, do not judge your emotions." Preparing for Brian's birthday, I'd been relentlessly upbeat–ice cream cake, new clothes, coordinating decorations for his room. Suddenly I realized I was denying the sadness enveloping me, trying to push around it, avoid it. I left the hospital abruptly that day, came home and sat in my study, hugging Brian's big red corduroy dorm pillow from Longwood. Tears flowed freely but gently, then the sadness left me, and I was free to plan the party and enjoy it.

But there was never enough discussion with Brian's brothers and sister and Curt about their fears and hope and pain or the impact this long ordeal had on their perceptions of themselves and their world. Sooner or later this volcano of suppressed emotions in the family unit had to erupt.

When we asked the social worker at Mount Vernon to suggest a family counselor to us, we found that there was no one they could recommend. After considerable research, we decided on a licensed clinical social worker whose office is near us in Springfield. Mark Rutkowski would become essential in helping us deal with the tasks ahead.

On the physical side of things, the hospital staff was well prepared to assist us in analyzing the physical modifications required in our home before Brian's return. Physical therapist Mary Beth Ireland and occupational therapist, Rosemary Fleury, visited the house in early November. Brian's mobility issues were easily managed in the hospital setting now, as his judgment had steadily improved, but mobility presented a whole new set of challenges when seen from the point of view of home. Brian was walking more in his therapy sessions and had regained almost normal movement in his legs, but injury to areas of the brain stem had impaired his sense of balance.

To imagine why Brian could not walk unassisted, stand straight and stretch your trunk from side to side, forward and back; consider how your body compensates and keeps you from falling in any one direction. That subtle bodily mechanism that all of us take for granted was not operative for Brian. If he leaned in any one direction unsupported, he would fall like a log. We thought his movements within the house would have to be in the wheelchair. As we began confronting this challenge, we considered looking for a single-level house; our split-level seemed impossible.

Rosemary and Mary Beth helped us to analyze more carefully, pointing out, "Actually Brian does better on steps than he does on flat surfaces." We determined that adding an additional well-bolted handrail on each section of stairs would allow him to move up to the bathroom or down to the laundry room with relative ease. He should be able to accomplish his shower unassisted if we added sturdy grab bars above the bathtub and purchased an inexpensive shower chair and a hand held nozzle.

Entering the house in the wheelchair could be accomplished with the addition of a ramp coming up the patio to the back door. Brian could be pushed or wheel himself through the carport and enter the kitchen this way. We had the ramp constructed with high siderails, so he could also use it to practice his walking.

Fortunately all our doorways measured large enough to accommodate the wheelchair.

The physical changes were easy and relatively inexpensive, but as always, the emotional changes were more of a challenge. The shifting of space for family members to accommodate Brian's return proved to be loaded with feeling, especially for me and my daughter Sheri. The middle bedroom upstairs had accommodated the young boys and the small bedroom had served as my office since I moved my typewriter there to compose a letter to Kaiser Permanente a year before. The large bedroom in the sub-basement and the bathroom on the lower level had been Sheri's domain since Brian left for college. Having just graduated from high school and begun a job, she was in many ways leading an adult life and valued her "private suite."

Now as we looked at how we would accommodate Brian, it was clear that she and I would be the losers of living space in the move. The younger boys would shift to the basement, an idea that pleased them, vacating the middle bedroom for Brian. But Sheri would have to move to the smallest upstairs bedroom, cutting her space by one third, and I would give up my office, my quiet space that I'd come to cherish.

If either of us had been more aware of our feelings, we might have sat down and discussed our resentment and anger, accepting it as part of our humanity. Releasing the negative emotions could have enabled us to go ahead with the moving process in a good spirit. But as it was, negative feelings were suppressed. We were "supposed" to be delighted. People would ask about Brian and say, "Isn't that wonderful that he's coming home after all these months!" and it was, but those pesky emotions would not dissolve without recognition.

One day in November, when Sheri had not met the deadlines set for getting her things sorted and moved, everything exploded. I shouted at her for not being helpful, and she attacked me for being too demanding. In an instant, we were almost ready for physical battle. The potential for hurt was significant that day, but we backed away as we both realized what was happening. We were angry at Brian and the situation, but the only place we could let that anger out was at each other.

Fortunately, our first session with the family therapist was scheduled for the following week, a safe place to air our fears at last. I surprised myself by stating that I was worried about how we were going to schedule showers upstairs every morning, a good example of displaced anxiety! Danny worried that Brian would fall when he was at home. Eric wondered if he would have to stay home to take care of his brother. Mark soothed some of us, drew others out and occasionally we engaged in brainstorming about how a particular issue might be resolved. Kaiser-Permanente agreed to cover the cost of this counseling for several months. The recommendation of the psychiatrist who had talked with Eric helped.

Rehabilitation patients at Mount Vernon Hospital often transition into an affiliated outpatient program called BRIDGE. The acronym stands for Brain Injured Daytime Group Extended. BRIDGE is designed to provide integration of treatment with community living and, as its name suggests, serve as a transition from hospital to life in the community–job, school, family, independent living. A proud accomplishment for many BRIDGE clients is the ability to recite what BRIDGE stands for. Dr. G. and the inpatient staff recommended Brian for BRIDGE, beginning in January 1987, and we learned that Virginia Medicaid would continue coverage. A hospital van would pick Brian up at Springfield Mall at 8:30 each weekday morning and return him at 3:00. We would be responsible for driving him to the Mall, four miles from our home. I decided on a three month leave of absence from my job at Hogan & Hartson, so I would be able to drive him. I considered myself lucky, since another mother I knew had driven a distance of 20 miles each way to deliver her son to BRIDGE before the van was available.

We were grateful for the existence of this established day program. Countless stories circulate among members of the Head Injury Foundation of survivors being discharged from intensive treatment to home with no transitional program and the resultant stress of such an abrupt ending.

In December, six months since Brian had really begun the process of accepting what had happened to him and of forging a new identity, we continued to prepare for the coming transition. I brought him blue jeans and grey corduroys to replace the gym shorts and sweatpants, routine attire in the rehab unit. Brian smiled his approval, then he agreed to go with me again to the Chapel. He moved easily to the bench this time. I read the 23rd Psalm, "The Lord is My Shepherd, I shall not want..." then Romans 8, "Nothing can separate us from God's love..." feeling inadequate. He became weepy, "All of this because of one stupid mistake; sometimes I think I'd be better off dead." The thought does not frighten me, because I've been there, but I'm not there now. I *hold* him, *feel* with him, and *know* deeply and surely this too shall pass. He admonishes me, "It seems like you're always preparing me for the worst." I wonder why he feels that way. He says, "It's hard to think of myself as head-injured–has a negative connotation. It seems I'm marked for life." The moment saddened me, but it signified a milestone for Brian on the path toward self-understanding and acceptance.

On Brian's second visit home, we were more courageous and expansive in our plans. He arrived at 10:30 a.m. I asked if he wanted to go down the two short flights of steps to his sister's room on the lowest level, the room he and his brother had formerly occupied. "I'd love it!" he said. Curt was resistant to the idea, thinking he might not be up to this much moving around. But we agreed it could be tried, with adequate support. We were awkward, getting in each other's way. I moved the wheelchair down the steps after him, crashing about. He negotiated both sets of steps carefully and deliberately. His presence in the house was consuming, larger than life, his body sturdy, solid, thrilling!

In the lower level bedroom, he sat on the bed next to Sheri and tumbled over on her, like a toddler. She responded warmly. We showed him where his dresser drawers were. He was intrigued. Baseballs, softballs, red-clay stained socks from that long-ago construction site job, stacks of old letters, his high school yearbook. He sat for over half an hour, shuffling through things, groping for the pieces of his past. He found a picture book with spaces for writing answers to questions, My Book About Me, filled in at age 5. He went through it page by page.

We took him to Mass with us. I was anxious–what if he got weepy, what if he had a too-sudden bathroom urge, what if people stared, what if he was "inappropriate" in any way. We decided on a seat by the side door. He insisted on sitting with us in the pew rather than on the wheelchair. I could hardly contain myself during Mass as he stood, knelt, placed his hands on the pew in front of us, looking so much like a regular guy, except for a front-on view of his face, with its misshapen jaw, droopy eye and trach scar. Several people greeted him before Mass, many others, especially singers from the folk group, after Mass. I am full to the brim. I feel like Zorba the Greek and want to *dance*!

Later in the day, when we were preparing to take him back to the hospital, Brian was weepy. Sheri, Eric and Danny remained with him at the table, not running from his grief. We gathered in the kitchen, in a circle with Brian to pray. He led us into the Prayer of St. Francis, "Lord, make me an instrument of your peace..." Electricity and warmth flowed around the circle, the spirit of a loving, living God within each of us as we recognized our ability to grow and learn with Brian.

• • •

Dr. G., in a rush of sentimentality, said at a December meeting, "We can discharge Brian on December 23rd, so he can be home for Christmas!" Somewhat hesitant to admit it, I spoke with considerable conviction for a small delay, "Couldn't we wait till about a week later? Christmas is hectic enough." Agreement was reached on a discharge date of January 10, with Brian to begin BRIDGE on January 3rd to assist with the transition.

We planned for him to be with us on Christmas Eve, but he must return before midnight, like Cinderella. Fairy godmother Medicaid says no overnights, or the family must pay the $250 hospital bill for that day. Our Christmas Eve tradition is beef fondue. We knew his chewing was not yet normal, but we decided instead of changing the menu for the whole family, we would prepare meatballs for him to cook in the hot oil. We didn't plan for coping with his judgment on the matter. He speared a piece of the chewy sirloin and cooked it in the pot. When he put it in his mouth, Curt and I insisted he could not have it. "Leave me alone!" he challenged as he clamped down on the meat, determined to eat it. Scott, brown eyes flashing, supported him emotionally. Curt and I protested, "He'll choke!" Danny ran away from the table in distress. Eventually the piece of meat is given up. Conflict subsides, we coax Danny back to the table, we recoup.

The high point of the evening was Brian standing tall and robust at the kitchen counter, dressed in grey cords and a blue plaid shirt, drinking carbonated apple juice in a toast "to Christmas–to family." My heart leapt at the sight of him, it was as though he had returned from the dead. The evening was filled with opening presents and family chitchat, pleasant, joyful, peaceful. We were forewarned that the hospital locks up at 12:00 midnight. Curt drove Brian back to the hospital, arriving at about 11:56, just in time to meet the hospital's "Cinderella" deadline.

Christmas day we picked him up again. This time we prepared for the meal differently. Turkey minced for him, mashed potatoes, sweet potatoes, all manageable foods, made for a smooth mealtime. He, Scott and I were sitting at the table after dinner. Brian picked up a carrot and took a bite, more testing. I looked at Scott, he looked at me. A mutual unspoken decision–we would not intervene, just wait. Brian held the carrot in his mouth a few minutes, then decided he could not, in fact, chew it. Taking it out of his mouth, he said, "Thanks for letting me work that out myself." One of many tests to come, but we were all making progress as 1987 began.

.5.

COMING HOME

*"It is only by risking our persons from one hour
to another that we live at all."*

—*William James*

Life is risk. Someone said, "A harbor is a safe place for a ship, but it's not what a ship is made for." The head injury survivor and his family are faced with constant and complex risk assessment. Protected from risk, the survivor remains childlike, unaware, and dependent. But one result of the injury is poor ability to "self-report," so the dangers of additional physical injury and emotional pain are ever present. During the months of Brian's inpatient rehabilitation, some risks were considered acceptable by the rehab staff and others were not. Often in the last half of that year, Brian had declared his intention to *walk* out of Mount Vernon Hospital; Chris Wade, his primary nurse, wanted to be sure he did just that. Still Brian's balance was not sufficiently improved for him to do any walking without hands-on assistance. Even at that, there was some risk. Chris is petite, 110 pounds; Brian, close to 165 and several inches taller than she. So Chris had to secure permission to walk Brian out the door. Dr. G. decided the positive effects outweighed the risk. Walking out that door would be a boost to Brian's self-esteem and provide a dynamic closure to Chris's year of dedicated work with Brian on the rehab unit.

His room at home had gradually assumed a new identity. Working there, painting, hammering nails in the border around the new carpet, I remembered the various transformations of the bedrooms. In 1966 this room belonged to Scott and Brian, tiny boys of three and a half years and 18 months, as the small room next door was made ready for Sheri's arrival. I pictured myself, swollen belly, sitting on the floor, refinishing a chest of drawers for the daughter about to be born. The one about to arrive now is yet another offspring. He is still Brian, but another being also, one who has lived through an unfathomable ordeal, to live a life that will be forever different from that which might have been. Only God can see where that life will lead him and all of us. If we could glimpse the creator's plan more readily, assessing the risks would be so much easier.

We had completed the physical changes required for Brian's homecoming. The grab bars were installed in the bathroom, the shower chair purchased, the ramp on the patio in place. I carved out a tiny corner of the sub-basement for my desk and typewriter. Sheri consolidated her belongings into the small upstairs room, but had begun looking for an apartment with friends.

January 10 dawned brisk and full of promise. We had gradually brought home all the items from the hospital room, Brian's "other home" for over a year. That morning we packed up the remaining odds and ends, magazines, little gifts, a board game of unknown origin, cards and letters received after the <u>Washington Post</u> series. Chris gave us last minute instructions about medication and reminded us to schedule appointments with the endocrinologist and ophthalmologist.

Brian had been convinced that he could not shower adequately without the hospital brand of soap, so he hoarded a supply. "We've got soap at home, Brian," we told him, but since it seemed an important matter to him in the transition, we allowed him to pack a dozen of the small bars, a compromise from the 40-50 he had accumulated. At one point Brian stood with his hands against the wall, "frisk 'em" fashion. Scott jumped to the cue, running his hands up and down his brother's torso, "He's clean!" No contraband soap! In addition to the soap, the hospital gave us a week's supply of Attends, disposable underwear that Brian still needed at night.

As the last item was packed up, Brian, dressed in his new clothes and wearing the cowboy hat we brought him from Montana, sat down in the wheelchair and propelled himself enthusiastically to the elevator that would take him down to the lobby for the last time. Chris said, "I've got a surprise for you, Brian, when we get downstairs." There, he and Chris began their farewell. He stood up and placed his hands on her shoulders. She walked backwards, supporting him carefully as he walked out the front door. When they reached our car, they embraced through tears; Chris said, "Don't forget to wear your seatbelt." Someone quipped, "She's still telling you what to do!" With the wheelchair placed in the back of the wagon and Brian in the front seat, we drove around the circle, past visitor parking, and into our new life. No longer would we have the hospital staff to decide which risks to take. We would learn to walk a fine line between what Brian wanted to do and what was acceptable risk from our point of view. We would also have to consider the impact of each situation on the rest of the family. We remembered Peter Patrick's sensible admonition about the survivor being "treated like such a miracle recovery that it becomes impossible to reintegrate him into the family" and treat him like a regular guy.

Some of the adjustments to be made were the result of Brian's "institutionalized" behavior. At the hospital, many people were responsible for his daily routine. Meals arrived miraculously on a regular schedule; a therapy was scheduled to fill each hour of the day. It had been a long time since he lived in the give and take of the family or participated in any of the normal routines of a 21–year–old.

In his room that first night, we tucked him into the full size bed, pushed firmly against the wall to reduce the risk of his falling out. Again the newborn stage came to mind, when I made periodic trips to hover over the crib to see if the baby was still breathing. But I slept peacefully through the night.

In the morning around 8:00, we heard a THUNK. Rushing into his room, I saw Brian curled up on the floor, grinning sheepishly. He explained, "I was trying to get the urinal." We'd left it on the dresser, three feet from the bed. He'd moved out of the bed purposefully and was crawling to the dresser when the dog, Katrina, came in and licked his face enthusiastically, toppling him from his hands and knees position. The following morning, he looked surprised when I walked into his room; then he told me,

"I saw you come in and thought, 'What's Mom doing at the hospital in her robe?' Then it came to me, I'm home!"

That first Sunday morning provided one of the first lessons in risk assessment. Scott was home from Blacksburg for the weekend. At breakfast, Brian was transferring from his wheelchair to a kitchen chair and lost his balance, falling to the floor, on his behind. No harm done, but we all felt our anxiety level rise. Scott, sitting closest to him, decided to let him get up alone. Curt and I agreed in theory. Brian started to pull himself up, lurchingly. But again his balance failed him. He lunged off to the side, head aiming straight for the corner of the sewing machine. Scott was the only one in a position to stop him. We shouted, "Scott!" just at the instant he too realized the theory could only be carried so far. He grabbed Brian's arm and pulled him back a millisecond away from impact.

We were solicitous those early weeks, following him when he left the wheelchair, which was used only on the ground level of the house.

He objected to this shadowing, but we insisted that it was necessary till we felt more confident of his judgment. He learned to announce his intentions, "I'm going up to the bathroom," and one of us would come to walk up behind him. Gradually, as we watched him grip the handrails carefully and choose his steps deliberately, we stopped this practice, allowing him to navigate the house alone–another step in our progress.

With his morning shower, the pattern was similar. Curt assisted him at first, carrying the shower chair to the bathroom, helping him into the tub, adjusting the water for the shower, and helping him to get out and dry himself. The bathroom was just too full of hard, slippery surfaces and lethal looking corners. But one morning as Brian came out of his bedroom and commanded, "Get me my robe and my chair," we decided the servant role did not suit our lifestyle. So we watched for signs that he could manage his shower alone. Within a few weeks we were convinced that Brian had learned the pattern of using the grab bars and compensating in this new environment and could be trusted to handle the shower himself. We decided to leave the chair in the shower during the day. There were a few minor mishaps and many shouts for help when the mysteries of the temperature control on the faucet frustrated him. "My robe and my chair" became family code for situations when Brian's behavior was a bit imperious.

Part of his work during his last months at Mount Vernon Hospital included washing his own clothes. So I resisted my motherly inclination to do it for him when he came home. Since he needed both hands to make his way down the two half flights of stairs to the laundry room, someone carried the laundry for him. But later in the year with the help of a laundry bag, he found he could complete the whole process himself. He felt good about doing it alone, most of the time, and we knew resentments were less likely to build up if we reduced the areas where he was dependent on us.

At the hospital, breakfast and lunch had been served on schedule. As with the robe and chair, Brian inquired, "Is my breakfast ready?" as he made his way down to the kitchen. We discovered during the first month that Brian could be self-sufficient at the morning meal too. Instant oatmeal was his favorite menu, and with a few instructions he could handle the measuring cup and the hot water in the microwave.

During the first months home, we decided to tolerate Brian's less than desirable eating habits. Brian added crushed saltines to nearly every menu offered him, chili, stew, split pea soup. Then he stirred it methodically till it became an obnoxious looking glop. Typically this stirring process continued until the rest of us were finished eating and until the food was cold. As other members of the family left the table, Brian would head for the microwave to reheat his bowl of "mortar mix," as it was later dubbed by his brother Eric. A few months after his discharge from Mount Vernon, he was admitted again overnight for the surgical re-alignment of his jaw. Now that he could eat more normally, we pushed him to at least modify some of his routines.

In March, Brian needed some new canvas shoes. It was time for an outing to the shopping center, his first "public" appearance other than Sunday Mass. We picked Herman's because they had a sale on high tops. As we pulled into the parking space, he said, "I feel a little embarrassed." I suppose he meant embarrassed by his dependence on me, but I didn't ask. We talked about situations that might come up, physical obstacles or encounters with sales people. We agreed to be patient with one another, calling it a "patience pact." We shook hands and headed for the stores.

In the crowded store, our first obstacle was benches lined up in front of the shoe display, the space too narrow for his wheelchair. After we'd found a position where Brian could look over the shoes, he chose a pair to try. Just as he was ready to point out his choice to the clerk, sudden toilet urge. Nothing in Herman's, the clerk suggests we try J.C. Penney's, "They have an elevator." Off we went at high speed. We didn't make it. The possibilities for a thoroughly frustrating moment for both of us were avoided. The patience pact worked. I threw my coat over his lap to hide his embarrassment, and we wheeled full speed toward the car. I felt for him, with him, but did not slide into pity or desperation over the incident. Leaving him in the car, I went back to pick up his shoes. On the way home, we problem-solved, recognizing the need to know the location of the men's room at all times. We also decided to keep an extra urinal in the car for emergencies. We used the "patience pact" on many occasions those early months.

The most emotionally loaded issue between Brian and myself, one that dragged on for many months, was his occasional incontinence at night. We used the Attends for the first few weeks, but the home atmosphere provided a strong incentive for him and for us to eliminate their use as soon as possible. About half of the time, he was able to use the urinal during the night and in the early morning and remain dry. The first few times his bed was wet, I took the sheets off while he was in the shower, washed everything and remade his bed while he was at the BRIDGE program. I wanted to spare him the embarrassment, and I knew he was trying. But given the still inadequate function of his short term memory, he would not remember that the bed had been wet, and he would resist taking ordinary precautions, like avoiding liquids in the evening.

So, heartless as it seemed, I began to insist that he take the sheets off by himself before he went to the shower and deliver them to the laundry room before he left for BRIDGE in the morning. I would usually wash them but leave them on top of the bed till evening, so he would have the benefit of visual evidence when it was time to decide on evening liquids. Some mornings, he would insist the sheets were only a little damp and they would dry themselves. His definition of "a little damp" and mine always differed, and many battles ensued. Brian's sense of smell is severely impaired, a fact that further complicated this issue. His neurologist eventually prescribed imipramine for him, which improved his continence and consequently improved our relationship.

Neuropsychologist Peter Patrick, who worked with Brian at the hospital and was again part of the team at the BRIDGE program, insists, "Living is the best therapy there is." With that in mind, Brian's adjustment to living at home with his family was the best therapy he had during the year of 1987. But a normal life is not confined to the family home. For this first year, the BRIDGE program provided structure, respite, balance and a sounding board for us. It was, however, a low-risk and consequently low-growth environment for Brian.

BRIDGE is structured as a three-month program, but frequently participants will complete the cycle two or more times. Brian continued for four cycles, the maximum, throughout the year of 1987. Unfortunately, most of the therapeutic activities at BRIDGE failed to motivate Brian. He seemed to feel he was doing the therapists a great favor by spending time with them.

The quality of adjustment for a brain injury survivor depends on how well he is reading himself, but the artificial environment of the hospital and programs like BRIDGE, in spite of good intentions, often shielded Brian from real-life experiences needed to improve his self-reading. On the other hand, BRIDGE provided outings into the community which were the best part of the program: swimming at a county recreation center, bowling, trips to the shopping center, rides on the subway.

Such ventures into the outside world were preferable to the unacceptably high risk of having him at home all day, sitting with the TV or playing solitaire, the fate of many who are discharged from intensive care back to their world without any transitional assistance.

The BRIDGE activity which did engage Brian's commitment was physical therapy with Buffi Smith, for that was progress toward walking, and in that session, Brian worked hard.

Brian's most consistently stated goal was to walk again. This was not surprising, since his pre-accident self-image rested strongly on his physical appearance and athletic abilities–a baseball player since elementary school, a wrestler in high school, hiker in the Shenandoah mountains, golf and frisbee in college. For a long time, he believed the wheelchair to be his only real problem. If his college girlfriend wasn't coming to see him as often as before, it must be "because I'm in this wheelchair." He believed that the only reason he couldn't get a job or drive was the wheelchair. If he could walk, life would be as before.

From the beginning of Brian's awareness of his body's limitations –" That's incredible, I can't walk!"– about half way through his year as an inpatient, we frequently advocated more actual walking as part of his therapy plan. After being repeatedly and patiently told that walking itself was not the best therapy, we acquiesced but always found the official theory hard to accept. Because Brian moved with stiff, robotlike motions, much work in physical therapy was designed to improve the tone of his trunk and leg muscles. This was considered more important than the actual walking. The neurological reasons may have been sound, but nevertheless, the logic of the approach always eluded us. As one who walks frequently for exercise and enjoys the sense of well-being that comes from the rhythm and movement, I couldn't see why endless repetition of the walking motion wouldn't have been beneficial, neurologically and physically, aside from the fact that it was what Brian wanted!

But we deferred to the specialists on this matter and learned to downplay the importance of the walking issue with Brian, suggesting to him frequently that he learn to live with the wheelchair as a necessary means of getting around and apply himself to improving his cognitive skills. I read him stories of people in wheelchairs shooting baskets, winning races, and heading corporations. He never bought it.

At home, we tried various things. We encouraged him to use the wheelchair ramp to practice walking. For a while, I had him pushing *me* around the block in the wheelchair, so he could walk accompanied and supported, while in a superior position. A friend brought him a trampoline with a stabilizing bar. We purchased an exercycle and considered a treadmill. Curt tried walking with him, on the patio or on the driveway. Nothing seemed to last more than a matter of days. He would set a goal and then forget to pursue it. If we reminded him, he'd be angry with us.

About midway through the BRIDGE year, they began allowing him to use a walker to get around the facility part of the time, but because he was still quite unstable and not the only client at BRIDGE, they often insisted he use the wheelchair for safety and expediency. In community outings, battles were fought because Brian didn't want to take the wheelchair, and the staff could not give him the one-on-one support necessary to walk from the van to the shopping center and back again. When we met with my sister's family in Pennsylvania in July for a day at the amusement park, Brian balked at using the wheelchair. He was unable to consider the needs of others in such situations. We allowed him to risk as often as possible, but one day as he walked, without the aid of his walker, the four feet from the front of the car to the post at the corner of the carport, he fell, fracturing his leg. Frustrated as we felt when this happened, it could not be used as a reason to further limit his risk-taking. Considering all he'd been through, a broken leg seemed little more than an inconvenience.

Two other subjects that seemed to elude our best efforts at progress during the BRIDGE year were vocational issues and driving. In one period of the BRIDGE day, a counselor led a group of people with brain injury in vocational exploration. The goal of this group was for participants to identify their work history, their ideal occupation, some of the obstacles that might prevent them from performing in a particular job, and setting up some realistic vocational goals for themselves. Brian was able to remember most of his work history, essentially unskilled work while a student: dishwashing, construction, installer at Sears Automotive Center, sales clerk at a T-shirt shop. His dream goal was still very vivid to him, an Air Force officer and possibly a pilot. After four sessions of BRIDGE and countless discussions on this topic, he was beginning to let go of that notion, but just barely.

On such vocational issues as this one, we all sidestepped the truth in our exchanges with Brian, which was ultimately a no-growth position for Brian. It came up quite often in my discussions with him. Not wanting to hurt him, I would say something evasive. Because Brian's perception of interpersonal exchanges was often very acute, he usually confronted me when my words did not match my expression or body language. Finally, I had to be honest with him about my feelings, although still sidestepping the issue, "Brian, I have too many mixed up feelings to talk to you about this. You'll have to discuss it with people at BRIDGE." I don't know what kind of evasions they used!

Driving was another issue that provided endless frustrations.

Brian made us the scapegoats because he felt confined to BRIDGE and home. "Why won't you let me drive?" he badgered us. "I could get a job if I had a car." Perhaps taking him to the Division of Motor Vehicles and having him take the eye test would have been a good reality check. The snag in this plan, however, was the possibility of his passing it! Passing the eye test only would have qualified him to renew his license, but that left out any assessment of his response times or other driving related skills. Vision tests at the hospital showed him right at the edge of driving eligibility. More recently, procedures have been put in place to assess a person's driving potential after an injury like Brian's, but at that time there were none.

Someone else suggested allowing him to get behind the wheel and try driving with one of us beside him, so he would have the benefit of that first-hand experience. Neither Curt nor I were willing to try it, and no basic evaluation of driving potential was included in the BRIDGE program. One day in October, however, Brian tried his own approach to risk evaluation.

We had just decided it was time to trust him alone for more than the usual 20 minutes. Planning to spend some time with his mother in Florida, Curt needed a ride to the airport. We decided to leave Brian alone for the 75 minutes I would be gone. I wrote down for him the time of my expected return, 2:45. After dropping Curt off, I returned home ten minutes early. I noticed Brian's walker sitting by the sidewalk and wondered if he had found a friend to take him to the grocery store. He had been frustrated that our plans for the day didn't include driving him for his groceries. "Good," I thought, "he is learning to be more independent in getting his needs met."

I went into the house to see if he left me a note. Nothing. I returned to the front yard to look for more clues. My eyes gradually wandered to Dabney Avenue as it slopes toward our driveway and saw an awesome, heart-stopping sight–Brian at the wheel of his sister's "new" Oldsmobile. He had found the keys and taken it for a drive. The car had been a hot topic of conversation around the house in recent days, Brian being very impressed with Sheri's new acquisition. Brian saw me and careered uncertainly toward the driveway, missing the mark slightly.

I looked at him with unbelief, then anger, then disappointment. Once he was safely in the driveway, the only reaction he saw from me was rage. "How dare you! What a stupid, irresponsible thing to have done! We trusted you to be alone for a while and you've done this." He looked sheepish and handed me the keys, but I kept hammering away at him. Then he retreated into the car, locked the doors and laid down on the seat, shutting out his mother's angry voice and stern face. I retreated into the house to cool down and realized that my response might have been "inappropriate," if understandable.

Later, when I returned to the car, unlocked the doors and asked him to please come in the house, he was repentant and tearful, "I'll come in if you promise not to yell at me!" I promised and helped him inside. He told me then how scary it was, when he realized that he was not driving right, could not judge the closeness to the cars parked on the side of the road, "so I just stayed in the middle." He apparently had not ventured as far as four-lane, heavily traveled Keene Mill Road, but had driven around the subdivision for quite some time. He had also planned very carefully to be back before I was due home at 2:45.

I pointed out to him, calmly, that he had endangered himself, others who might have been driving or walking, and his sister's new car, definitely not a good risk to have taken. I tried to acknowledge the feelings that led to this action: the need to be more independent, the feeling of being trapped at home so much of the time. We discussed the possibility of his driving again in the future, but only with the proper safeguards and correct conditions.

The next day I discussed this traumatic, but by now humorous, incident with Betty Bradley, the new director of the BRIDGE program. She suggested having him write down how he felt when he was in the car, so he could pull back the memory of his feelings of uncertainty by reading it in his own words. I gave him a piece of paper, "Write about how you felt when you were driving, Brian." He wrote, "I felt free like a bird must feel when it flies. I felt fear from a retribution or distress from the thought of you finding out. Fear from the law! Puzzled at my erratic driving, but FREE, really FREE!" If the emotional content of my anger was equally memorable, maybe it was not so inappropriate after all! We have had no more such experiences, but we are careful not to leave car keys accessible.

At the end of his year at BRIDGE, Betty asked Brian to write up something about his experience in the program. The essay he wrote gives a glimpse into the slow growth of his self-understanding during that year. Here's part of that writing:

WHY BRIDGE

A little over one year ago, I came home. Back to the house I had lived in for twenty years. My mother gave me a big hug and said, "It's good to have you back at home." "I'm glad to be out of the hospital, but now they want me to go to this thing called BRIDGE. It's some silly class. Just something else to get out of."

Basically I didn't want to go, but they said everybody goes, so I figured I would also. At the end of my first session, they told me most people go for two sessions, and I went bananas. Then at the end of my second session, I just figured I had another, so I went. Then when the third session came to an end, I was lost. I thought that was the most you can have, and that they would graduate me.

Then I had one of my rare brilliant ideas. I figured if I have improved this much after three, what would happen after four, so Betty said she would love to have me back.

My attitude now towards BRIDGE is a complete about-face from what it was before. In my fourth session, I remember looking at some of the new people with distaste. Then I stopped. I'll bet I was like these new people when I first started. All of a sudden they didn't seem so bad.

When Brian began the fourth session at BRIDGE in the fall of 1987, the challenge again began to shift to us. What would Brian do every day when this last session ended? We had frequently brainstormed with staff about possibilities. The next step for many in the Virginia Rehab system was Woodrow Wilson Rehabilitation Center, a vocational training center in Fishersville, VA. WWRC provides job training for approximately 50 occupations in the building trades, health care, food service and business to people with a wide range of disabilities. We had visited the center long ago, when Brian was still in the shock-trauma center in Baltimore. Now we were advised to submit an application but were disappointed to find out that the waiting list was one year.

We learned of the newly organized Teamwork, a creative blending of the Council for Exceptional Children and the Council on Aging. Teamwork connects senior citizen volunteers with disabled young people to help them find employment. We contacted Teamwork and were referred to Warren Schmidt, a personable retiree from the U. S. Geological Survey. Several job trials were set up for Brian during the latter part of the BRIDGE year. At a nearby nursing home, he worked at filing in the office, and wrapping silverware in napkins for food service. After Warren met Brian, he accompanied him to these job sites, to get to know Brian and give him occasional feedback.

On one occasion Brian spent a few days painting the wainscoting at the nursing home, but his impaired vision and mobility made this a tedious undertaking. As Warren told him with a smile, "I don't think you'll be able to do this for a living, Brian!" But at least Brian was experiencing himself in some real-life settings, "normalized environment" in rehab lingo.

Delivering the mail at Mount Vernon Hospital was conceived as another job trial. Brian's sociability sabotaged this task. Having spent 13 months at the hospital, Brian knew and loved many of the nurses, therapists and other personnel. Delivering mail, he would invariably stop to chat with many people along the way. His vocational counselor tried to use the mail delivery to teach him to complete a task within a certain time frame. He had to deliver the mail to the hospital and be back in time for his van ride back to Springfield. After several weeks of this, Brian was "fired." The concept of this task as a job trial did not click; the social experience was more important every time.

Much like our experience while Brian was still in shock-trauma, the problem we faced at the end of BRIDGE was "What next?" as Brian continued to have trouble with his "jobs." The bridge began to look more and more like a long pier, leading to nowhere. What can he do; what programs are available; how will they be paid for?

The Brookers, another family in the Virginia Head Injury Foundation, especially well-supported by their insurance company, had, after reaching the end of the same "pier," found placement for their son Matt in Galveston, Texas, at an innovative head injury rehabilitation facility called Transitional Learning Center or TLC. Since we had friends from Springfield currently living in Fort Worth, I planned a trip to Texas. Rosalie and Scott Shipe, who had been with us the day of Brian's accident in 1985 would drive me to Galveston for a look at TLC's program.

Russell Moody, the son of wealthy Texas businessman Robert L. Moody, sustained a traumatic brain injury in 1980 at the age of 19. Like all the rest of us, Russell's parents experienced the agony of their son's injury and the frustrating search for a program to bring him as far as possible. However, Moody had a distinct advantage over the average parent; he controls a significant portion of the business and real estate in Galveston. After learning all he could about the most successful programs, Moody financed the development of Transitional Learning Center in 1982. This state-of-the-art rehabilitation center helped his son Russell reach a high level of recovery and continues to be one of the best models in the country.

Community integration and outreach are especially effective at

TLC. Clients have maximum real-world involvement: jobs at banks, libraries, grocery stores, and other businesses, so that their problem-solving classes and therapeutic exercises can be readily connected with their daily experiences. Whatever the limitations and abilities of the TLC client, a place is found where growth can take place. TLC has its own bus to provide transportation to work and recreation, in addition to a contract with a cab company for reduced fees for clients with limited financial resources.

As impressed as we were with the facilities at TLC, it was not a viable alternative for Brian. There was no way we could afford the $550/day price tag. I did write to Kaiser-Permanente to describe this facility and ask if they would like to fund Brian's participation, but I fully expected the negative response which I received. For residents of Texas, TLC rehabilitation is funded by the state agency for rehab services. If Brian could have become a legal resident, perhaps by living with our friends temporarily, we might have found a way to do it. But such solutions seemed too convoluted; besides the geographical distance between Galveston and Virginia was a disadvantage. So TLC was crossed off our list of viable options.

At this stage our Virginia Department of Rehabilitation Services (DRS) was of very little help. Brian was assigned a counselor at the local DRS office, presumably to provide ongoing support, once the BRIDGE program ended. But from the time of his initial interview in the fall of 1987 till May of 1988, the turnover rate for counselors was phenomenal. He had four different caseworkers in seven months, making it quite impossible to build a working relationship.

Work Adjustment Training, a DRS program that had been suc-cessful with several of our Head Injury Foundation friends, was another suggestion. But in a meeting with the director, we were told, "Brian is not eligible, because he has not yet made enough progress to benefit from this program." Without a program of any kind, it seemed he would regress, so how was he to become eligible? Brian, whose hearing loss is a significant detriment in any group discussion, missed most of the details of this meeting, but picked up the negative tone. As Warren Schmidt, Brian and I left that meeting in Alexandria, I was filled with anger and frustration, more than at any time since the days when Brian was in a coma. The anti-tipper bars on Brian's wheelchair were being repaired, and as he wheeled down the hall after the interview, the chair tipped over backwards, Brian's head hitting the hard tiled floor. Fortu-nately, the only consequence was a large bump, but if Warren hadn't been there to help us recoup after this mishap, I think I might have collapsed on the floor with Brian and wept.

On a more sober day, I decided to stop projecting the worst; we would manage, one day at a time. No program or job training was available for Brian at the end of BRIDGE. His DRS counselor suggested a course at the community college, which sounded like a good "real world" experience, maybe a little too "real." Could he find his way around campus? Was there any transportation besides Mom and the LTD? Could he really advocate for himself in a classroom, requesting special seating arrangements so he could hear? Could he remember what he did hear? I contacted the Learning Disabilities counselor at the college and learned that her caseload numbered close to sixty. I didn't have the heart to begin to explain Brian's needs.

All things considered, though, we decided it was a risk worth taking. He was enthusiastic about the idea, so we registered him for a basic math class in the spring quarter. DRS would pick up his nominal tuition, since it was considered a step that would help prepare Brian for Work Adjustment Training. Unfortunately, he broke his leg a few days before this class was to start, tipping the scale against it for the time being. The broken leg also eliminated an adaptive swimming class we'd found for him.

FRIENDS

A few of Brian's college and neighborhood friends courageously stayed with the process of his rehabilitation for a long time. The June after his accident, about 15 young people came to a party at the hospital, organized by Karen, a neighborhood friend since she and Brian were toddlers. Karen was a faithful friend for a long time, but finally decided she needed more feedback, "Why don't you call me sometimes, Brian." With little response from him, she could not sustain the relationship. At the time of his discharge from Mount Vernon, we planned a party for friends and MVH staff who had become like family. Many came, and we hoped some would stay in touch with him for the long haul, but by January 1988, two and a half years after the accident, contact with pre-accident friends was minimal. Inevitable and understandable as this fact was, it was nevertheless a painful reality for us and for Brian.

When he first came home from the hospital, he thought everything would be like old times, especially with his oldest friend in the neighborhood, his "blood brother." He imagined him coming up through the woods behind the house and the two of them going out the way they did as teens. But it was not to be. For a while Brian called him regularly, and he would come by every few months, but it was never the same. Slowly, painfully, Brian let go of his old friend and accepted the end of that relationship.

His girlfriend from Longwood visited and encouraged him all through his stay in the hospital, but during the year in BRIDGE, she knew she had to be getting on with her life. The following year she was married. A young woman we all came to love, she still calls him once in a while. We're not sure which is kinder, to call him or to stay away, but we know how good we all feel when she calls!

Mark Holland, his most loyal male friend from Longwood College stayed in touch by letter for many years and managed to visit occasionally. He went on to graduate from law school and was married in Richmond a few years ago. We attended the wedding with Brian and wore our "pleased to be here" expressions, but such occasions tend to be bittersweet reminders of our losses.

In what seemed a void as we began this risky period with no program and few social contacts for Brian, some bright lights came along. Brian had become friends with a pretty young woman named June Friedman while he was in the BRIDGE program. June, then 27, had suffered a brain aneurism three years earlier while a college student. Like Brian, June used a wheelchair to move around and had worked through a long tedious process of recovery. But she was a bit farther along than Brian in several respects. Having already participated in Work Adjustment Training, June had worked at several volunteer jobs. She was nearly ready to move on to a paying job. After BRIDGE she and Brian wrote to each other regularly. She encouraged him in many ways that only a peer can do.

Visiting with June and her mother, Brian and I were impressed with the collection of completed jigsaw puzzles that adorned the walls of her bedroom. Brian wanted to decorate his room similarly, so we began buying puzzles. His vision limited his effectiveness with the puzzles, but it proved to be a satisfactory family activity, filling in some of the empty time, and it kept several of us busy with him on many winter days and evenings.

At a wedding reception, one of the first social events Brian attended, he met Danny Gallagher. Danny, now in his 30's, had survived a serious injury in a car accident and was now operating his own landscaping business. Danny took Brian out several times, swimming and to a disco, sort of a good ole' boy relationship that delighted Brian. Arriving in his big blue truck, Danny would burst energetically on the scene, "Git off your big behind and let's go!"

Ken Bounds, a retired FBI agent and long-time family friend, took a personal interest in Brian. Ken is a six foot three former athlete, who walks with difficulty himself because of his arthritic knees. In addition to knowing Brian as one of the neighborhood kids, Ken, a volunteer at the Rec Center, worked with Brian during the BRIDGE program's adapted swimming sessions. Ken came for Brian and walked him around the block many mornings, or sometimes they drove to the high school where Ken worked as a substitute teacher. Ken would ask the school to leave the gate open, so when he and Brian arrived at 8:00, they could drive across the field and park close to the track, a perfect place for more practice. Ken also picked him up occasionally and took him to a basketball game or other sports event at the high school. This was therapy that money could never buy.

A month or so after the end of BRIDGE, we decided to investigate another innovative program in Pennsylvania. Al Condeluci, a speaker at the annual conference sponsored by our local Head Injury Foundation and Mount Vernon Hospital, was gaining recognition for his community integration and independent living program for brain injury survivors. He worked with United Cerebral Palsy Association (UCP) in Pittsburgh and had discovered many similarities in the needs and aspirations of both groups. In a telephone conversation with Al, we learned that his program was covered by Pennsylvania's Office of Vocational Rehabilitation (OVR), that state's equivalent of our DRS. Since I was a native of Pennsylvania, and my parents still lived there, funding might be worked out, if we could push the right bureaucratic buttons.

When we arrived at the UCP building on Centre Avenue, Curt and Brian waited in the car while I went inside. The young woman at the reception desk suggested I sit down in the activity room till she could contact the person who was to meet with us. I walked unprepared into a room of people whose appearance shocked me. Since Brian's accident, I had learned about relating to and understanding people who were "different." But here in this room were approximately twenty-five people with cerebral palsy, most of whose bodies appeared twisted into distressing forms. As my eyes darted around the room, I panicked and literally ran back to the car. Then I felt ashamed and amazed at the ignorance still within me. When I returned, I sat down to wait, reminding myself to see through the contorted body to the person within. With that thought firmly planted, I was able to converse comfortably with several people while I waited.

The physical environment in Condeluci's program was less agreeable than that of TLC in Galveston, and a February day in inner city Pittsburgh was dismal, but the program had many strengths. The day program held at the UCP center appeared to be similar to BRIDGE. And as a brand new client Brian would have to remain in the day program for an indefinite period till they could assess his needs and strengths, before moving into their most innovative programs, supported employment and independent living.

In our conversations with staff, we heard of excellent working relationships with the business community. Many employers leased space in their corporate environment for vocational exploration groups to meet. In this setting, they could meet company workers, observe different work settings, ask questions, and determine their own job-related goals. When it was time to place a person with disability in an actual job setting, a job coach provided one-on-one support till the new employee was able to be self-sufficient.

Another significant part of UCP's program was their Independent Living Rehabilitation Program (ILRP). We drove from the UCP center several miles through Pittsburgh to Shaler Highlands, a cluster of apartment buildings perched on a high hill. ILRP rented ten two bedroom apartments in the complex, each of which housed two of the program's brain injured clients. In order to be eligible for the apartments, clients needed a job or a day program, for which transportation was provided. Resident counselors, who lived at Shaler in their own apartments, had beepers and could be reached by phone any time they were needed. Oversight by the counselors included a visit in the early morning and late afternoon to see if everybody's day was moving along on schedule.

In their newsletter the program was described, "Residents live, shop and recreate along side other citizens. This concept tends to deemphasize differences and promotes a greater sense of similarity."

In ILRP's statement of philosophy on community living, we found some challenging assumptions:

— People with disabilities are intrinsically valuable individuals, capable of contributing to the communities in which they live.

— All individuals are capable of growth and development.

— All individuals are unique and develop at their own pace.

— Individuals with disabilities should be provided with the <u>least restrictive environment</u>.

— All persons must be afforded the <u>right to risk</u>.

The statement goes on to stress that residents, their family members, and their funding sources must accept the inherent risks involved in the pursuit of independent living.

We worked for weeks to get Brian into this program, because of its many pluses, but ultimately failed on funding. Pennsylvania OVR was understandably reluctant to pick up a person whose rehabilitation was really the responsibility of the Virginia rehab system. At one point in the process, the director of the Pittsburgh region wrote to his equivalent in the Virginia system to request funding from Virginia for Brian to attend a program in Pennsylvania. This request was denied. We considered how we might pay for the program ourselves, less expensive than TLC, but ultimately decided this was not feasible. Finally we withdrew the application.

Brian's 23rd birthday was coming up. Warren Schmidt, visiting with Brian in early April, listened thoughtfully while Brian discussed his expectations for a birthday party. Glancing sideways at me, Warren observed, "Sounds like a lot of work for someone." I decided the next day to turn the planning totally over to Brian, since this event had a high motivational factor. He spent a day writing and rewriting the invitation, making his handwriting as neat as possible. I drove him to the library to make copies. Back home he planned his guest list, trying to balance friends and people from Mount Vernon Hospital and BRIDGE. His list included Chris, his primary nurse from Mount Vernon, therapists from BRIDGE, and the hospital van driver. He collected addresses and made out envelopes. This really developed into "occupational therapy," since planning and organizational skills are frequently a problem after a brain injury.

The next day I suggested he write up a plan for food and drink for his party. He wanted cold sandwich meats and something hot. We decided on a pot of chili. Then we went over the necessary ingredients, and he wrote them down. It was decided that I would drop him off at the grocery store, while I had lunch with a friend. He planned to inquire at the deli about party platters.

When I picked him up an hour later, it was clear he had had a satisfying shopping trip. Grinning proudly, he reported, "I bought apple juice, orange juice and Seven-up for punch, and a fresh pineapple and strawberries to put in the punch." In the car on the way home, he marveled about another topic, "While I was waiting for you, I saw all these girls in mini-skirts; it was enough to make my head swim!"

At home he showed me the brochure he got from the deli clerk, with pictures of the available party platters. We looked it over together and decided on "The Hostess." As is often the case, it would have been far easier for me to make the call to place the order, but this was something he could do himself. After a recent meeting with his audiologist, we'd acquired an adapter for his telephone. This was a perfect opportunity for him to practice. After locating the number on the brochure, I wrote it out for him in larger numbers. I touched the monitor button on the downstairs phone to see how it would go. He did well until she asked which platter he wanted to order. He had forgotten which choice he made a few minutes earlier, and faltered. "Uh, uh, was it the Hostess or the Buffet Supreme?" The clerk's voice showed a trace of impatience. I decided to intervene, running up to his room and pointing to the correct one on the brochure. He continued, "Yes, it's the Hostess that I want. I would like to pick that up on Sunday morning. Thank   you."

Did I make the right choice to intervene? I was never sure. When he came down the steps, he thanked me, but in some similar instances he was angry. If I had let the conversation go on, he would eventually have made a choice and it would have been OK. The choices, after all, were not dramatically different, and no real risk was involved here. In addition, if he had fully experienced embarrassment in the conversation with the clerk, it may have impressed him with the necessity of writing such things down.

On many days, Brian had nothing to do aside from his meals. Not surprisingly he gained weight. I had to detach from this "dead" time and keep up my own agenda. Watching television was not particularly satisfactory in spite of a device purchased to help him hear better. I did not consider this a great loss, and neither did he. He resumed a pre-injury pastime, reading Louis L'Amour novels. He had a collection of 60 paperbacks, but the print was too small for him at that point. However, the library stocked large-print editions of L'Amour books. This proved to be an excellent self-directed activity for Brian, exercising his mind, his vision, his memory, and feeding his spirit. He often shared with me passages that particularly touched him, usually about the heroic adventures of L'Amour's frontier men and women. In many ways, Brian too was a man on the frontier.

In early May, we placed an ad in our parish bulletin, asking for working opportunities for Brian, paid or unpaid. Our older children had attended the parish school for years in the 1970's and Brian remembered many of the teachers. The librarian responded to our ad, requesting Brian's help in replacing labels on books during the remaining six weeks of the 1987-88 school year. We grabbed this opportunity for him to work on his attention span and writing skill in a comfortable social environment. Warren Schmidt agreed to accompany Brian initially to provide on-the-job support. Brian enjoyed the work and the opportunity to talk with his former teachers, who treated him like a returning hero. But when school was over in the middle of June, the job ended. The librarian wrote up a positive evaluation of Brian's work, attitude, and potential. This experience became the first post-accident item on the resume we would prepare for him later on.

Although the library job was a positive work trial, Brian could not see himself working in a library on any long-term basis. It always seemed to us that the truly inspired job idea would somehow tap into the interests and skills of the pre-injury Brian. Nothing tried so far had even come close.

In the spring and summer weather, I always imagined him learning to operate a ride-on lawn mower. My father, whom Brian idolized, had worked as a groundskeeper for a large estate in Pennsylvania. "What do you think, Daddy?" I asked him when he visited, "Could Brian be trained to run a small mower?" He pointed out that these vehicles usually had a "dead-man switch" that would stop the motor instantly, if Brian fell or if the mower tipped over. My father is a practical man so when he thought it over and said, "Yeah, I think he could do that," it seemed worth pursuing. Naturally Brian liked the idea. One of his most satisfying summer jobs as a high school student had been the Youth Conservation Corps at Turkey Run Farm, a recreation of an 18th century Virginia farm. Warren figured his vision and his judgment would be issues, but agreed the idea had some merit. Warren contacted the Fairfax County Park Authority, which employs hundreds of people in its network of parks and recreation centers here in Northern Virginia. The answer was negative, liability insurance cited as a reason, but they did suggest we write them a brief letter describing Brian's strengths. They would try to find something for him at South Run Recreation Center, a newly constructed facility just four miles from us.

In my first phone conversation with the director of South Run, my hopes were dashed when he said, "We were thinking of using him at the front desk to answer the phone." When I told him Brian's hearing loss minimized his effectiveness on the phone, he said, "Then I don't think we have anything for him." Because he sounded kind and genuinely interested in helping, I called him back the next day to see if Warren and I could come talk to him about the work they had and where Brian might fit. He agreed to see us.

Director Bob Foor was willing to take a chance. He decided Brian could assemble brochures and keep the information rack stocked. In addition, he could work with the maintenance man washing tables and windows. Brian would work four hours three days a week as a volunteer. He started at South Run the middle of July in 1988. We reached a compromise about how he would get around at the center. He used the walker most of the time, but kept the wheelchair in their storage room for special situations. I worried about him staggering around the office, falling, disrupting things, but this was needless "mother worry" and exactly the kind of thing I knew I had to stop! Summer workers at the center included a number of attractive young women and Brian quickly made new friends.

During the BRIDGE program, Brian had been constantly urged to write things down to compensate for short term memory problems. For the most part, he remained unconvinced of the need to do this, causing endless frustration for us and for BRIDGE staff. But within weeks of beginning his new job at South Run, he had a convincing reason to use this technique. When he found he couldn't remember the names of his new women friends, he went to one of the older employees and asked her to go over all the names with him, so he could *write them down!*

After a month on this job, he received a letter from Woodrow Wilson Rehab Center that he had been moved up on the list and would be admitted to their program in Fishersville in September. This was four months in advance of the original one year estimate, and it was frustrating to have him accepted for training just as we'd found something on our own. We believed that our inquiries with the Pennsylvania rehabilitation agency expedited his application.

Among many brain injury survivors in Northern Virginia, the assessment of Woodrow Wilson's brain injury program was poor, and we were only too aware of this reputation. We decided to make a conscious effort not to take any prejudices with us when we drove Brian down for his initial interview. One obvious difference at WWRC is the presence of more men on the staff. With each person we met, a case manager, an occupational therapist, a speech therapist, a vocational counselor, questions were asked more directly to Brian instead of us. Ten minutes at the end of an hour interview was our time to modify or add to Brian's answers. Not that this approach had been totally absent from previous meetings with professionals, but more focus on the client himself seemed a step in the right direction, so we were hopeful.

Realizing that Brian's absence would free up a lot of my time when he went to Woodrow Wilson, a residential program, I decided to sign up for courses at Trinity College, again beginning in September. Some "letting go" was necessary, so we made an active decision not to be too frequently in touch with Brian's progress at WWRC. Some things he would have to work out alone, and we needed a rest.

In early September, we helped him pack up his clothes, his laundry bag, his cassette player, and moved him to Fishersville. The two things I did write up to pass on to his case manager at WWRC were his volunteer work at the school library, his recent experience at South Run and the possibility of operating a ride-on mower. The Assistant Park Manager had written, "Brian has a wonderful attitude and it is contagious. We have enjoyed working with him." It seemed logical that staff at WWRC might pick up on the rapport already established at the Rec. Center and find a way to train him in skills needed at the Center, leading eventually to paid employment for the Park Authority. The WWRC setting seemed a logical place for a tryout of his potential on a ride-on mower, since the complex has plenty of lawn to be maintained. Then I let go and concentrated on my courses and my relationships with Curt and the other children.

Brian stayed at Woodrow Wilson till the early part of February, with several weekends and the holidays at home. WWRC's mandate is vocational exploration, training, and placement in jobs for people with a variety of disabilities. But in Brian's case, the exploration went on for months, without any discernible result. Very little effort was made to work with the Park Authority, to the best of my knowledge. And no trial was ever given on a ride-on mower. It seemed instead that WWRC had a certain routine drill everyone had to go through. Brian's psychological denial and poor insight into himself limited his ability to participate fully in the process. But, it seemed the system had very little room for creative or innovative thinking; and limited opportunity for the hands-on contact with the working world we'd seen in Galveston and Pittsburgh.

To be fair, they did give Brian a brief job trial at a local library and offered him library assistant training, one of their established programs, which he turned down, much to our disappointment. In WWRC's discharge summary mailed to his local DRS counselor, they concluded that Brian was untrainable at this point. He could go back to his volunteer job.

For reasons known only to WWRC, we were never able to receive a copy of records kept during Brian's stay there or of his discharge report. We wanted to know what skill evaluation and job trials they had conducted and the specific results. Unable to obtain this, we had few facts to evaluate. All we knew was that six months and forty nine thousand DRS dollars later, paid for by the state of Virginia, Brian was no closer to vocational discernment or training than when he left his volunteer job at South Run to move to Fishersville.

However, we did see growth in Brian in several non-vocational ways. His roommate at WWRC was a young man paralyzed from the waist down since birth. Knowing him and being aware of the personal care assistance he required helped Brian put his own disabilities into some perspective. He also became more aware while at WWRC that his parents had worked hard at being his advocates in the rehabilitation system, a fact that had not penetrated previously.

But if vocational goals were not met for Brian at WWRC, one accomplishment towered over all others in his mind. Under the guidance of physical therapist Steve Walden, he learned to walk without the wheelchair, always his first and foremost goal. Steve worked steadily with him, training him to use two canes with arm supports. When he came home from WWRC in February 1989, the wheelchair was parked in the carport, where it collects dust, a fact that Brian loves to point out.

I felt free like a
bird must feel when
it flies. I felt fear
from a retrobution,
or distress from the
thought of you
finding out, Fear
from the law!
Puzzled at my
erratic driving,
but <u>Free</u> really

<u>Free!</u>

Letter from Brian to his mother during his recovery.
(See pages133-134 for more letter samples.)

· 6 ·

LETTING GO

*"There are two lasting gifts we can give our
children; one is roots, the other is wings."*
–Unknown

Letting our children go out from us to live their lives, make their own mistakes, pursue their own dreams, is as important in the rhythm of nature as the death of leaves in October and their dramatic re-emergence in the spring. Necessary as it is, letting go is seldom easy. Our children come to us utterly helpless. They must be fed, diapered, bathed, loved. We may complain about this awesome responsibility, but being needed by another human being is a gift in itself. Just as Mom and Dad learn the joys of being needed, this tiny emerging person learns the word "no." Translate that, "I'm not always going to do things your way!" And that's only the beginning.

When our oldest son Scott was preparing for college, I was finding it difficult to let go of some of the usual concerns. Would he make the "right" kind of friends? Would computer science be the best major for him? And what about this coed dorm? A friend gave me a copy of an anonymous poem called "Letting Go." Since the words of the poem seemed to express the ideal, a family tradition was born. As Scott packed his trunk, I tucked a framed copy in between his socks and the notebooks. When Brian left for college in 1983, he too received a personalized copy.

Letting Go

To a dear one about whom I have been concerned.
I behold the Christ in you.
I place you lovingly in the care of the Creator.
I release you from my anxiety and concern.
I let go of my possessive hold on you.
I am willing to free you to follow the dictates
of your undwelling Spirit.

I am willing to free you to live your life
according to your best light
and understanding.

Brian, I no longer try to force my ideas on you,
my ways on you.
I lift my thoughts above you,
above the personal level.
I see you as your Creator sees you, a spiritual being,
created in the divine image, and endowed
with qualities and abilities that make
you needed and important—not only to
me but to the Creator's higher purpose
I do not bind you. I no longer believe that
you do not have the understanding you need
in order to meet life.

I bless you.
I have faith in you.
I behold Jesus in you.

                                        –*Author Unknown*

As I prepared the bedroom for Brian's return home from Mount Vernon Hospital in January 1987, I found his copy among the miscellany he brought home from Longwood College two months before his accident. As I read the words, they seemed a mockery. The process of letting go had been well under way, when it was violently interrupted that fateful morning on a lonely Maryland road. Now he was returning to us in a state of childlike dependency. Would letting go ever be possible again? Were the rules radically different for a son whose life process had been so dramatically altered?

On a Monday evening in the early part of 1988, during the time when we were most concerned about finding another program for Brian, we listened to neuropsychologist Dr. Peter Patrick at one of the regular support group meetings of the Northern Virginia Head Injury Foundation (NVHIF). About 25 of us, many parents of brain injury survivors, sat in a large circle. He challenged us, "Most of you let go of your children once, when they went off to college or moved out of the family home? Why is it so hard to let go again?"

"That's easy, Peter," I volunteered. "Before, he was a regular kid going off to college–now he can't walk, can't hear, can't see very well, can't remember, and barely understands what happened to him!" The answer seemed self-evident. I was not yet ready to consider being able to let go of Brian for the second time. But now, nearly four years later, Brian has grown in self-awareness, and we are hopeful that he will have an opportunity to live independently. He must have his wings.

The fact that we can see this as a possibility is directly related to the many hours we've spent with other families and survivors in the past six years. When Brian was still in a coma, meeting other survivors five to six years post injury provided a viable image of recovery. Now, many of those young men and women have reached the next step. Some have jobs or meaningful volunteer work and their own apartments. In short, they "have a life," though not the life they would have without their injuries.

Hearing the mountains and valleys their parents had crossed gave Curt and me courage. On days when the stress seemed overwhelming, letting off steam to another parent restored my sanity. During 1991 and 1992, answering many calls from family members at the office of the local chapter of the Head Injury Foundation, I've been able to provide a similar outlet to others, an outlet that can be a matter of life and death. For those who remain isolated with their challenges, the outcome can be tragic.

A chilling example of the worst possibility came to my attention about a year after Brian's accident. On July 12, 1985, just two days before Brian was injured, The Washington Post ran a story, "Alexandria Mother Slays Son and Herself." The son had survived a head injury three years earlier in a motorcycle accident; his unpaid medical bills had climbed to $500,000 and were growing at a rate of $50,000 a year. The family had just lost a $10 million lawsuit brought against the manufacturer of the helmet their son wore. The next day, according to the Post, "the mother took the family revolver and emptied it into her son and herself." In the fall of 1991, we received a call from a mother. "My son killed himself in July," she related. "He had a head injury about five years ago, and we had never heard about your support group." It is not difficult for me to imagine the despair felt by these people. If we had not met people who had coped successfully, we might have fallen into similar despair.

The stories we hear from members of the Northern Virginia Chapter of the Head Injury Foundation have common threads, familiar to us from our experience since July 1985. Most of us have an anger that can burst instantly to the surface when a conversation touches on a raw nerve. For one family, it's the thought of the youth who chased their son through an alley, forcing him into the path of the oncoming car that nearly killed him. For another, it's the doctor whose faulty drug prescription caused their son's brain damage (they won their lawsuit). For one mother, it's the emergency room staff who inexplicably sent her toddler daughter back home after a fall, saying she would be OK. For many others, the villain is an impersonal insurance company that refused to understand, and pay. Or the professional, often a neurosurgeon, who said, "There is no hope," or "If he survives, he will be a vegetable."

For the persons in our group who have sustained a brain injury, the anger surfaces on different issues. "They told me at... I'd never be able to walk again," or work, or speak, or drive, or learn. "My brothers and sister have moved away from home, have their own place, and I'm still here." "I want to work, but I can't get a job." Or for those who sustain a "mild" injury, "They sent me home from the hospital and said I'd be just fine!"

And for a few severely injured persons, the negative predictions such as we'd heard in the trauma unit come true. Approximately two per cent of those who survive traumatic brain injury remain in the lowest levels of the coma scale for years, in a "persistent vegetative state." The son of one of our members died recently after eight years of severely limited life. This family, like us, fought hard to secure the best rehabilitation for their teenage son in the early years after his accident, but eventually they knew he would not return to meaningful life; they had to let go. He lived his last years in a nursing care facility, where his basic bodily needs were met and he received some stimulation.

In our Northern Virginia Chapter, we know of approximately 25 people with brain injuries who live in nursing homes or require total care from their families at home. We are certain there are more that we don't know about. The options for these survivors are pathetically limited. Insurance companies regularly threaten to stop paying for the already inadequate nursing home care. Families adjust to mere maintenance for their sons and daughters or struggle constantly to secure care that includes such stimulating activities as outings to a shopping mall or a park. The patients in the recent movie, Awakenings, had survived encephalitis and remained in a state analogous to level one or two of the Rancho los Amigos scale. Similarly, "low-level" survivors who exhibit limited response to their environment experience occasional "windows" of meaningful response. Jeff, a young man injured in a 1978 car accident at the age of 17, lives in a nursing facility. His mother relates, "We took Jeff a letter from his sister at Christmas. You could see the excitement in his eyes as he scanned the letter."

Mild brain injury represents the opposite end of the spectrum. When we are inclined to believe Brian's recovery might have been complete without the additional trauma of the cerebrospinal meningitis, we gain perspective listening to persons who sustained a "mild" brain injury. Unconscious for only hours or a few days, they are often discharged from the hospital, looking well and believing their injury had no lasting effects. But soon, thinking problems and personality changes affect their ability to function in their former job or in their family relationships.

Because they look just as they did before the accident, these brain injury survivors have problems different from Brian's. Friends and relatives often find it hard to believe there is an organic reason for the changes they see in the injured person. Theresa Rankin was a junior at San Diego State University when the Porsche driven by her boyfriend careened off a cliff in 1977. She describes her early confusion:

> "After three weeks I was released from the hospital. Four months later I was trying to go back to college. After having always been an active and visible participant in classes, there I was, sitting in my spot and finding it <u>so</u> difficult to understand what the professor was doing, what he was saying! I couldn't grasp that words made a sentence, that a sentence made a concept."

Not until many years later would Theresa find professional assistance to help her name these experiences as subtle cognitive impairments that were the result of her brain injury.

Differences in functional abilities can sometimes provide opportunities for creative mutual support. One survivor has a tendency to speak too rapidly, words tumbling together, as a result of his injury. Brian, with his hearing impairment, recently asked John to please "slow down." John told me later, "Maybe I need to talk with Brian more; that forces me to slow down, which is what I need to do!" Brian Quigley, a 17 year old brain injury survivor, needed someone to be with him during the fall 1991 break in the BRIDGE program. Melissa Mills, injured 11 years ago and looking for a job, proved to be a sensitive, understanding companion for Brian that week, enabling his mother to continue with her job.

For us as Brian's parents, assessing the risks of the many stages of his mobility is another area where the support of other parents and survivors has been especially welcome. One mom and dad who have encouraged their son to drive again, in spite of the many risks involved, provided us with a model. If we kept in mind that we wanted a maximum degree of normalcy for Brian, it was easier to work our way through each stage. For instance, when Brian returned from Woodrow Wilson Rehab Center, able to walk at a reasonable pace with his canes, he was anxious to try out his newfound mobility. For our sake, he agreed to wear a bike helmet when he walked around the block alone till we felt more certain of his stability. In a couple of weeks, we were able to relax when he went out with his canes.

Letting go of issues related to Brian's physical safety seemed relatively easy to manage, our initial anxieties giving way to a workable trust, but issues involving his memory and altered perceptions of reality have been much more intractible. In these more subtle and complex areas, families find it harder to assist one another, and very little trained professional help is available when the survivor reaches the end of available rehabilitation.

Brian is jealous of his possessions, sometimes crossing the border into paranoia. He is the only one in the family who eats bran flakes. His morning ritual includes pouring a bowlful of cereal, peaked up like a volcano in the middle, then adding milk and allowing it to soak into a soft mush, usually creating some overflow in the process. This amount of cereal is more than the average serving, so he finishes a box quickly, but forgets just how much he has eaten. During one period, he accused other members of the family, sounding like Papa Bear, "Someone has been eating my bran flakes!" Finally, after numerous discussions, some reasonable and some loud, we encouraged Brian to keep his cereal in his room. That problem was solved, but frequently some other issue takes the same form—missing hearing aid batteries, pens, loose change, or laundry soap.

In addition to memory problems, Brian's bodily sensations are altered because of injury to his central nervous system. As he puts it himself, "My body plays tricks on me." His awareness of this fact is growing, but occasionally he has created absurd explanations for what he feels. His neurologist prescribed imipramine for Brian during outpatient rehabilitation to help him remain continent, but for the last two years, he has not needed it, much to everyone's satisfaction. At one point, he experienced sensations that reminded him of the effects of imipramine. Curt took him to the neurologist, who explained, "Considering your injury, this is normal."

But Brian preferred to form his own explanation: his mother was sneaking imipramine into his food. He was obsessed with this idea for weeks. If I served him first at the dinner table, he would apply a line of reasoning that went like this: "Why did I get that particular spoonful of chili–you made it a point to give me that spoonful!" I would usually respond to these accusations with sweet reasonableness, "Brian, think about it, why would I want to do that?" only to dissolve into shouting when he persisted. "OK, I'll *never* serve your food again!" Of course, I would forget that resolution when we sat down for another "happy" family meal, and soon we'd be on the same merry-go-round again. One evening, the topic came up when just the two of us remained at the table. Tempers began to rise. I asked Curt to join us; I needed an arbiter. After Brian repeated his story, Curt decided on a more dynamic reaction than is his usual patient, laid-back style. "Brian, this is the damnedest, most ridiculous idea I've ever heard! I don't ever want to hear it again, do you understand me?" That particular topic receded, but the faulty thinking tends to enter into other problem-solving.

Not surprisingly, such behavioral issues are intensified by social isolation. A significant development for us locally was the beginning in 1989 of a recreation group sponsored by the Fairfax County Department of Recreation and Community Services, known as the Weekenders. When Brian is on his way to a Weekenders outing, (or a job) he has no time to monitor his laundry soap for signs of foul play!

One Sunday morning, the Weekenders planned a trip to King's Dominion, an amusement park two hours from us. Brian had been looking forward to this for weeks. Twice cancelled because of rainy weather, the trip was finally on. He needed a ride to the Springfield Mall by 8:30 a.m. to be picked up by a van funded by the Rec Department. Surprisingly, Brian suggested bringing the wheelchair. "We'll be doing a lot of walking," he said, as he put the chair in the back of the station wagon himself. When everyone arrived at the pickup point, six survivors and several people from the Rec Department, he asked if he should take the chair. Lisa Silverman, the energetic young woman most responsible for helping our sons and daughters gain access to this service, answered him, "Brian, you're going to be walking your feet off today! We're gonna tire you out; you don't need that chair!" The atmosphere was that of any group of young adults leaving for a day trip. In my car, headed back home, I breathed a sigh of gratitude and relief.

This is the way it should be, good-humored peers urging him to exert himself into a day of fun.

• • •

On occasion I have an opportunity to view an event from a different perspective. Survivors who willingly adopt a strategy of keeping a daily calendar or journal tend to be the most successful at re-exerting themselves into the community and being able to follow through on a task. Those of us advancing in age are well advised to adopt the tactic as well! I write everything down nowadays, probably obses-sively. If I drive anywhere in the sprawling metropolis of Northern Virginia, the directions are recorded on a card that rests in my lap, "left on Rolling Road, right on Braddock, etc."

Last summer, Brian had an appointment with his audiologist in Arlington. As we sat in the driveway, ready to go, I looked over my notes. Brian said, "That's interesting that you write everything down– Dad remembers the way." Later, when we had made a wrong turn and I referred to my notes at a stop light, he commented again, "That's pretty good, you know your deficits and compensate for them." I bristled, but captured the irony of the moment, as I responded, "Uh, well, no, it's not that I have deficits; it's just that it's the smart thing to do!"

• • •

When the survivor finds his own voice, learns to read himself correctly, and adopts the smart strategies as his own, he begins to take charge of his own recovery. The larger community, unaware of these heroic but wounded men and women, can better understand if they listen to the voice of the person who has survived a brain injury.

One vehicle that allowed survivors to find their voice was the yearly information conference co-sponsored by the Northern Virginia Chapter with Mount Vernon Hospital for survivors, families and professionals. In 1988, while Brian was away at Woodrow Wilson, a survivors' panel was planned for the conference, in addition to talks by several nationally known rehabilitation professionals.

BRIDGE director Betty Bradley and I met with five brain injury survivors to assist them in preparing five minute talks. Each of the young men and women selected for the panel seemed to have made real progress in taking over responsibility for their recovery and were actively involved in the community, employed or in school. At our first meeting, we posed some questions to each survivor. What happened to you? Where were the turning points in your progress toward self-acceptance and understanding? What are some of the coping strategies you use? What advice would you give to other brain injury survivors?

Knowing a thought, expressing it verbally and/or writing it out is a complex set of mental processes for anyone. For a person with brain injury, it is a skill slowly relearned, if ever. But we believed that the five persons assembled for the panel possessed unique insight into themselves and hoped to assist them in expressing that insight in their own words. During one-on-one conversations with each panel member, their answers to the questions were drawn out and recorded in the computer. With the printout in front of them at home, they could re-read their own words and think more about their answers before our next meeting. The process of working to prepare for these talks was a moving and educational experience for Betty and myself, for the panel members, and eventually for conference participants.

The self-understanding expressed by Tom Stumm was especially poignant and enlightening. Tom had been a senior engineering student at the University of Virginia at the time of his injury in 1982. The process of Tom's recovery paralleled Brian's in its length of time and complexity and in such details as walking, and short-term memory problems. Tom has never regained his ability to speak normally, but nevertheless is able to make himself understood by a patient listener. With people he's just met, Tom uses a word board, pointing to words he's trying to form.

When Tom gave his presentation at the conference, his words appeared on an overhead screen while he spoke at the podium. Here are some of his thoughts:

> Life was very hard for me the first few years, because I denied everything. I thought the things every one of my supporters was telling me wasn't true. I thought I was on another planet. I refused to live in the real world where real things happen. I would say to myself and to others, "I am not in the right body." Before the accident, a lot of the time my brain did what I wanted it to; it was very reasonable. For the first few years after my injury, I said simple things that I wanted to get done; the brain and body wouldn't let me do them. It was very depressing.

> How does one live in the real world and stop fantasizing? For some a change of attitude has to happen. The head injured person has to

live with what they have *today*. Many think in their own minds, "I was once real smart, so I should be able to do that now," or they think, "I will do what I want to do right now, in the way I want to." On the other side of the coin, some head injured people think, "I will never be able to do that."

If I didn't know that I had a brain injury, changing jobs from a civil engineer to a clerk in a library is pretty poor. Knowing that a brain injury has happened, to switch jobs from civil engineer to clerk is pretty remarkable. As a matter of fact, it is amazing!

I understand my deficits now. I hope that they will get better, but I have quit fantasizing and am able to live in the real world. Changed attitudes can come from the head injured person observing those around him. If they see other people around them succeeding, they will think that they can succeed too. Head-injured persons should think of themselves as winners!

Hearing what Tom had to say, we were painfully reminded that Brian did not yet have a comparable insight into himself, or at least we were not aware of any such insight, and neither were the staff at Woodrow Wilson, who had just discharged him as vocationally untrainable. In spite of my resistance to Dr. Patrick's comments about letting go, I knew that I was powerless to effect the growth of Brian's self-understanding. I decided not to again take up the task of searching out a program or a job for him. He was able to resume his volunteer work at South Run Rec Center, a total of eight hours a week. We would have to trust and see what came up with time and through Brian's own experience of himself. I concentrated on my coursework at Trinity College and sought to detach myself as much as possible from Brian's everyday ups and downs.

During the summer, Brian was assigned a DRS counselor who brought new enthusiasm to that role. Rhonda Woodward took the time to study Brian's file and, after meeting him, expressed disagreement with Woodrow Wilson's view that Brian's vocational potential was extremely limited. A paid position seemed critical to Brian's independence and self-esteem, so Rhonda recommended Brian again for Work Adjustment Training (WAT), the program considered inappropriate for him after BRIDGE ended. He began WAT in September 1989. Once again, we were grateful for some structure in Brian's day. Brian would be occupied four days a week, from 9:00 to 2:00, at the DRS center in

Alexandria, and transportation would be funded. Objectives set out for him sounded familiar: to improve memory for tasks, to identify realistic job goals, to improve ability to give and receive instructions from others, to utilize his calendar to keep track of assignments.

As part of WAT, another volunteer placement was found for Brian in the fall of 1989. He would now work at United Community Ministries, an Alexandria non-profit agency which provides emergency food, clothing, shelter for needy citizens, as well as referrals to other county services. Brian worked in their office Tuesdays and Fridays, transcribing information from application forms filled out by people seeking help. By observing him in this setting and receiving feedback from the people he worked for, his supervisor at WAT could assess his ability to complete tasks accurately, to accept direction, and to handle interpersonal relationships on the job. Wednesdays and Thursdays, he explored job related issues, practiced interview skills, and worked on the computer at the WAT offices. The position at U.C.M. proved to be Brian's most successful, long-term volunteer job. He continued with U.C.M. for a year, but when he completed WAT, no paying job was found, and DRS could no longer fund his transportation to Alexandria. A relationship that was successful for Brian and for U.C.M. ended.

In the spring of 1991, an opportunity arose for Brian. A few months earlier he had attended a job fair in Washington, one of several regularly held for persons with disabilities. He went to the job fair on his own, armed with a completed SF-171, Application for Federal Employment. He met a recruiter for the Air Force who was favorably impressed with Brian's potential. In April, she called to discuss a job in the civilian personnel office in the Pentagon for Brian.

We called Rhonda Woodward, his case manager with the Department of Rehabilitative Services, and Marianne Talbot, his case manager at the Head Injury Services Partnership (HISP), hopefully putting into motion the support systems that would turn this opportunity into a permanent placement for Brian. As his parents, Curt and I tried to be relatively detached, but we saw this as a major breakthrough. Brian was hired as a GS-4 for a six month probationary period.

HISP was able to provide funding for a job coach, a young man who would accompany Brian on the job for the initial weeks, assisting him with transportation and suggesting strategies for organizing the tasks that would be required. Once again, the physical challenges seemed the easiest to overcome. Brian could board the bus at the end of our street, and arrive at the Pentagon in 40 minutes. His job coach accompanied him till he mastered the route from the bus stop to his office, through the maze of Pentagon corridors.

We wondered if he would have the stamina to get up at 5:00 every morning, leave the house at 6:30, put in a full day and return home at 4:45. If these physical challenges were the sole measure, Brian succeeded. With a special alarm system for people with hearing impairments, he got out of bed on his own, showered, shaved, ate his breakfast, and left the house well-groomed and eager each morning. He set out his wardrobe for each week with enthusiasm. "Mom, would you look at these pants, shirts and ties and see if they match?" Curt helped him master the art of the necktie. He relished arriving home in the afternoon and having me ask, "Brian, how was your day at the office?"

"The real world doesn't cut you much slack," said Dr. Peter Patrick, speaking recently at one of our chapter meetings, referring to the attempts of survivors to make their way. "When an opportunity does arise, it must be managed," he continued. Brian's opportunity at the Pentagon was not well managed. Neither case manager had sufficient input to Brian's supervisor to give her insight into Brian's disability. The job coach, although competent and willing, was not sufficiently trained in working with persons with brain injury. Brian's supervisor lacked sensitivity. Brian himself lacked a sense of the reality of the situation.

No doubt each of the principals in this job trial would see things from a different perspective, but this is mine. This job represented one of the first times Brian experienced himself (and his deficits) in a real world setting. Part of the job involved a process of pulling personnel files and recording information about each file. His supervisor and his job coach had assured him that speed was not important, accuracy was. It was correctly determined that Brian could do that part of the job. A young man hired for the summer came in regularly to assist Brian if the file processing was backed up. Brian became acutely aware that what took him an hour to do, Harvey could accomplish in 15 minutes. So listening to his feelings instead of his supervisor, he would try to speed up, increasing the margin for error and frustration. When he felt frustrated, he lashed out at co-workers and his supervisor. On one occasion, when his supervisor stopped him in the hall after work to ask if he had written an end-of-the-day summary she had requested, he responded, "Don't bitch at me!" In his defense, Brian said, "She had already told me I was not going to get a permanent job, and it was after work hours!"

We attended several grueling meetings with case managers, supervisor, job coach and Brian over the course of the six months, but the end was in sight by the end of the fourth month. After five and a half months, Brian's job was finished. "Involuntary termination," reads the dispassionate government form. Much as we'd tried to keep our expectations on hold, it was a bitter disappointment for everyone. Perhaps the most helpful interchange on the subject was overheard at one of our support group meetings. Melissa Mills. told Brian, "I've lost three jobs in the last five years, before this job I just started." Brian laughed and observed, "So maybe you're saying that I've got two more to go!"

Intrigued by Melissa's words of consolation, I decided to learn more, especially since she now has found a very satisfactory job. Melissa, the daughter of a cardiovascular surgeon, sustained her relatively mild head injury at the age of 16 and was unconscious for a few days. With the help of private school and tutors, she completed high school three years later. She tried college, but in her words, "There was no support at that time and I just didn't fit in."

After a string of unsuccessful job tries from 1984 to 1990, in retail stores, restaurants, and one hospital, Melissa decided she could no longer do it alone. To the average person, Melissa looks fine. "People don't understand," she says, "They don't know that I have to concentrate all the time to succeed."

In contrast to Brian's experience, all the pieces were in place for Melissa. After canvassing possible employers, job coach David Klein of ICON Employment Services found an ideal opportunity for Melissa. Women In Communications, a trade association for women in media, needed a receptionist. When David told them about Melissa and her special needs, they were receptive and enthusiastic. David then spent a week at the job site analyzing the required tasks. He took pictures of the staff of seven, assembling a small album with names; then he suggested the staff wear name tags for the first few weeks. He prepared a folder of detailed instructions, made a labeled box for sorting mail. He instructed the staff, "If she asks too many questions, tell her to look in her book." Four months on the job now, Melissa is delighted with her new work environment. She says, "I feel like I am part of the world, part of life, instead of being an outcast."

In addition to an understanding employer and a thorough job coach, Melissa herself was fully ready to take advantage of this opportunity. Having felt the sting of many failures and conquered a drinking problem that began a few years after her injury, she had reached a point of clear-eyed self-understanding and self-esteem. The journey to that point is a long and complicated one for most survivors.

Brian's most dramatic progress began when he himself initiated a project through a chance encounter while he was still volunteering at South Run Rec Center. Bridget Wyrick was shepherding a group of four-year olds in Kiddie Korner, the Center's summer day camp program. Lined up in front of the water fountain, each of the children came to her to be lifted up to reach the stream of cool water. Brian, sitting off to the side waiting for his ride, his canes propped on the bench beside him, watched this little parade intently. "Why don't you put a chair beside the fountain? Then they could stand on it and get a drink without any help," he observed. Bridget smiled at him, "You know, you're right!" She introduced herself and the children to Brian.

The next time they spoke, he told her, "I've often thought of talking to school kids about wearing their seatbelts, but I'd need some help to do it."

"He knew what he wanted to say," says Bridget, "I told him I had some teaching background and maybe I could work with him. I was intrigued with Brian, and knew there was really a need for this!"

When Brian told me about his conversation with Bridget, I too was intrigued, but highly skeptical. I kept my doubts to myself, deciding to wait and see what happened next. Was this woman really going to follow through? And besides, Brian would probably forget the whole thing the next day. Wasn't this another bright idea that would fizzle before it got started? But Brian did remember and Bridget continued to remind him of his intention. When the subject came up repeatedly, I realized that Bridget might need some feedback from us, so I asked Brian to get me her phone number.

When we met, I knew she had the tenacity and imagination to see this project through with Brian. She asked if we minded open discussion of his drinking and pot smoking the night of the accident. "No, if talking about it can prevent others from making the same mistake, that would be wonderful," I told her. Still, I was anxious about Brian speaking to a group of teenagers. Thinking about it, I could find no reason for my anxiety, except the possibility of his experiencing rejection, the kind of worry that belongs in the "let go of it" column. Curt and I agreed that Brian might make a significant impact on high school students, so we gave Bridget an unequivocal go-ahead to help him put his idea into action.

At about the same time, we were again preparing a five-person survivors' panel to speak at the Fall 1989 NVHIF conference. This time Brian was scheduled to be on the panel, a perfect opportunity for him to try his speaking ability in an accepting environment. Betty worked with

Brian and two other panel members to put their talks together, while I worked with the two remaining panelists. I first heard Brian's talk when we met to begin rehearsing.

The first weekend in July of 1985, I was accepted into the Air Force ROTC. The second weekend in July, I had a car accident. The next thing I remember was a year later.

I can't remember any of that missing year. I can't remember my accident. I can't remember the night before, the year before, or the two years before. But five years before, I can. Maybe that's good, maybe that's bad. I say that because I can remember what I was like, and I know what I'm like now, and I don't always like what I see.

Like a wine, you're supposed to get better with age–something is wrong. A head injury is catastrophic and is almost like death. In fact it is the death of you as you were, and is the birth of you as you are. I often relate surviving a head injury to being reborn.

Why? Well, when you first wake up, you may not be able to walk; you may wet your bed; you may not be able to eat by yourself; you may not be able to drink out of a glass. I don't know what else, but you name it, and it's probably something you can't do.

But slowly you re-learn, slowly you become closer to your actual age. There is a birth of a new, but not always improved you. It may appear in a way that does not fit the old you. In my case, I've switched from a physical person to a mental person. For example, it's hard for me to trust my senses. My hearing is impaired; my vision is limited; I can't smell, and my feeling is decreased on one half of my body. I used to use my physique, my looks, my athletic prowess to attract friends. But now I don't have those, so I use my brain. And my brain attracts real, not superficial friends. My athletic friends don't come around anymore–I can't do what they can do. Life goes on.

It has been a difficult transition. There have been times I didn't like the change. I guess I still kind of long, mourn for that old Brian, that physical me, but when I look at it, I don't think I'd switch for a million bucks. Because the friends I have now like me for me, not for what I can do. Those are the friends that you want to keep all your life.

My next challenge is to get a job, to have a place to go and a chance to earn money, but most of all, to give me a feeling of accomplishment as I further my recovery and continue my new life.

I felt like a mother might feel hearing her son deliver a valedictory address. Brian had clearly made some giant steps in the process of his recovery.

When this public appearance was successfully completed in October of 1989, Brian was ready to start speaking to students. By November, he and Bridget had pulled together some ideas for a presentation to Driver Education classes at West Springfield High School, Brian's Alma Mater (Class of '83). We didn't realize the connection this project had to the pre-accident Brian till Curt brought home from Florida a cassette tape we'd sent to his parents in 1981. It included messages from all of our children. Brian, then a junior at West Springfield, spoke about his public speaking class. "Everything we do in there is fun," he said, with youthful enthusiasm. "You have a formula for your talks, which is CASC: Capture, Assert, Support and Conclude. You have to capture the attention of your audience. My public speaking teacher says that if you don't get their attention in the first thirty seconds, their brains go on a mental vacation." As Brian planned for his talks to students in the fall of 1989, the principles learned eight years earlier were clearly operating in his mind.

He knew how he wanted to capture the attention of his teenage audience. He would have Bridget push him into the classroom in the wheelchair; then he would rise slowly from the chair, with these words, "Did that look easy? It took me four years to do that!" During the remainder of his talk, Bridget helped to keep him on track by asking leading questions. That first appearance at the local high school was a strong beginning; students wrote to him expressing their reactions:

"I think you had a big effect on many of the students who listened to you speak. I hope what you said opened up some eyes and ears."

"It cannot be that easy to visit where you used to go to school before your accident. We watched a lot of movies telling us the dangers of drinking and driving, but meeting someone who has lived through it is a lot more effective."

"Having you talk to us shows us how things can affect us, even though teens usually think they'll be young and able bodied forever."

"You really convinced me how important seat belts are. It takes a lot of guts to get up in front of everyone."

"No one in the class will forget you."

"Your story made me believe that drinking and driving is not at all safe, and I swear I will never practice it."

"You are a very special guy and have a lot of courage. Never lose your sense of humor and keep smiling."

Brian and Bridget spent a day each at three local high schools in the early part of 1990, and in March, they were invited to travel to Richmond to speak at a teen health forum. That presentation was taped:

Brian: What do you think? Did that look easy? It took me four years to learn to do that!"

Brian's tone is impassioned.

Four years of non-stop work, four years when I could have been following the occupation that I had picked out.

Bridget: Brian, could you tell us something about yourself in July of 1985?

Brian: I just finished my sophomore year of college. I had plans to transfer to Virginia Tech, switch my major to mathematics and enroll in the Air Force ROTC. On the first weekend of July in 1985, I went down to Tech, was measured for an Air Force cadet uniform, and the second weekend in July, I fell asleep while I was driving. The next thing I knew was a year later.

Bridget: This is the way the accident was described in The Washington Post:

At 1:00 a.m. on July 14, after having a few friends over for a small party, Brian Rife and one of his best friends, Tom Kilday, 21, got the urge to go to the ocean.

An hour later, Brian put some towels, a shirt, a pair of pants and a bathing suit into his mother's 1978 Dodge Omni–with a

Virginia license plate that said MS RIFE–and headed for U.S. Route 50, the road to Ocean City, MD.

Brian drove, and Kilday sat in the front passenger seat. Neither wore his seat belt. The roadway was dry, but a light fog hung in the hot, sticky air. Kilday remembers stopping once at a 7-Eleven, where they bought potato chips and burritos. Then, Kilday said, "I went to sleep, woke up once to see if Brian was all right, then went to sleep again."

At 5:30 a.m., still 35 miles from Ocean City, Brian dozed off. The white-colored Omni drifted off the road, right at the point where the highway begins to curve sharply to the left, according to the police report.

Brian woke up just as the car hit the shoulder, still traveling 55 miles per hour.

"Tom!" Brian screamed.

A second later the car sideswiped a light pole, which broke away, and then hurtled down the embankment. It smashed into a utility pole, lifting Brian out of his seat and hurling him across the car. His head cracked into the right side of the windshield, right in front of Kilday. As the car began to flip over, Brian fell against Kilday and their legs became entangled.

The car finally stopped, upside down, about 400 feet from where it left the highway.

Photographs, taken by the state police and the Rife family, tell the rest: blood splattered on the corner of the windshield. Broken glass on the dashboard and the front seat. A Frisbee just inches from the open passenger window. A beer can, apparently from the wreck, resting nearby on the wet grass.

As they lay there, their legs wrapped together and caught under the steering wheel, Kilday remembers turning to Brian and asking, "Brian, can you hear me?" There was no reply, but Kilday said later he was relieved to see that Brian appeared to be unhurt, except for a trickle of blood from his right ear.

During the next 20 minutes, Kilday drifted in and out of consciousness several times, Kilday said. At some point, he heard the sound of footsteps and voices; he remembers nothing else until awakening in the Hebron Rescue Squad ambulance, whose crew had to use a harness to pull him and Brian from the car.

Within an hour of the crash, the ambulance arrived at Peninsula General Hospital in Salisbury, MD. Doctors quickly determined that Kilday's injuries were slight–cuts on his back and a bruised knee–and he sat at the hospital for four hours waiting for a ride back home. Brian, however, was still unconscious; the trickle of blood that Kilday had seen was evidence of a severe brain trauma.

Bridget: Were you drinking the night of the party?

Brian: That's probably an understatement. I was guzzling the night of the accident. The first guy showed up with a 12 pack of beer, the second guy showed up with another 12 pack of beer. By easy multiplication, that's about 8 beers apiece.

Bridget: Was anyone smoking pot that night?

Brian: Yes.

Bridget: Were you wearing your seatbelt at the time of the accident?

Brian: No.

Bridget: How do you feel today about seatbelts, Brian?

Brian: At that time, I never wore my seatbelt. I had five years of driving experience without wearing my seatbelt. I had two car accidents; I still didn't wear my seatbelt. Now, the car is not even out of the driveway before I've got my seatbelt on. I have a friend who has survived a head injury. I get into his car and he doesn't even start the engine till I buckle up. He won't say anything, he'll just sit there.

Bridget: Because you weren't wearing your seatbelt, your head hit the windshield?

Brian: Well, if I had been wearing my seatbelt, my head would not have hit the windshield, 95 percent chance I would be in the Air Force today, flying an F-15 over your head, but instead I've been stuck in that thing.

Bridget: How long were you in a coma?

Brian: The original coma, about a week, I came out of it, walking around a little bit, but my nurses and therapists would show me a picture of my Mom; I'd look at it: "Who's that?" They'd show me a picture of my Dad or my roommate in college. I didn't know who anybody was! Then after a few weeks, I got spinal meningitis. Big name, but all it really means is an infection in the brain that threw me back into a coma where I stayed for five months.

Bridget: Brian, what is that scar on your neck?

Brian: It's where I used to breathe –no, that's wrong– it's where the machine used to push air into me because I couldn't even breathe. I have another scar here on my stomach. It's where a machine used to push food into me because I couldn't even eat.

Bridget: Brian, are you going to get rid of those scars?

Brian: I thought about it, we actually went to see a surgeon. At the last minute, I decided no. I'm not ashamed of those scars. Those are battle scars, mark of a strong competitor. I'm here, I won and I'm happy to be here.

Bridget: Brian, how is your hearing today?

Brian: I wear this little thing in my ear, it's called a hearing aid. My left ear is completely deaf. I take the aid out when I go to bed at night. The most heavenly thing in the world, not to hear a sound. Alarm clock, I don't even hear it.

Bridget: How is your sight?

Brian: It's funny, everyone in here, even with my glasses on, has four eyes. I can see every single person, but I couldn't tell you when anyone blinked. There is no clarity to any of it.

Bridget: How is your smell?

Brian: I always thought my sense of smell was all right. One day

I was at home by myself. My younger brother came home from high school. The minute he walked in the front door, he said, "Brian, what's burning?" I said, "What the hell are you talking about!" He went into the kitchen. Sure enough, Mom had left something on the stove, and it was boiling away.

Bridget: What were some of the things you had to relearn?

Brian: Talking, hearing, seeing, everything.

Bridget: Brian, when do you use this wheelchair?

Brian: Only when I come to one of these talks. It sits in my driveway folded up, collects dust. I want to see this chair sitting in the carport, collecting dust, because I want the feeling of knowing that I don't need it any more.

Bridget: Brian, would you show the group how you can walk.

At this point, Brian walks across the front of the room, staggering, lurching, grabbing desks or chalkboard to steady himself, but he always makes it.

Brian: Funny, I often have women open the door for me. When they see me with the canes, immediately they think, "poor guy," then open the door just out of niceness. I'm a guy; I'm supposed to open the door for women! I want to say, please let me open the door for you.

Bridget: Brian, you want to become independent. Can you share some of the ways you work to gain your independence?

Brian: My mother has me do my own laundry. The washer and dryer are downstairs; my bedroom is upstairs. There is no chute to drop the clothes down. They don't even bring the basket downstairs for me. I have a big bag I put all my dirty clothes in. I throw it down the first flight of steps, hold on to the handrail and go on down. Pick up the bag, throw it down the second set of steps. When I finally get down to the laundry room, I sort darks and lights. My eyes are not good enough to read the measuring cup, so

I don't know how much detergent to put in. My solution, I buy those one-shot detergent packets.

Bridget: In conclusion...

Brian: I have sat here and talked to everybody about the hazards of an automobile, of drinking, driving, drugs. But if one of you, just one of you listens to me and wears your seatbelt, I am a success. If more than one of you, or many of you, wear your seatbelts, those are the things that dreams are made of.

Dear Mom Saunders
I wish to thank
you for ~~the~~ the ~~~~
marine t-shirt ~~that~~ you
gave me. I'm very
happy with the
way it ~~f~~ ~~happy~~ fits me. l
Also hope that you
and Dave have not
worried too ~~at~~ ~~~~
much about me.
with much love B aren

Letter from Brian to his grandparents during his recovery (1986).

To the Springfield Council of the Knights
of Columbus,

I would like to Thank you for
enabling me to go to camp this
year!

I had the chance to see alot
of familiar faces, faces I only see
down at Camp. The high point of my
week was seeing my X-primary
Nurse, Chris Wade!

I have some limitations because of
Head Injury. Because of these I took
it easy, until the last day!

I signed up for Earthball + then
soccer! Needless to say, Earthball,
which is Rugby with a 6-foot round
ball, caused me to twist my ankle!

I didn't Realy hurt myself. "aint
nothing but a Thing!"

Thank you, again

Sincerely,

Brian Rife

Letter from Brian to the Springfield Council of the Knights of Columbus (1993).

.7.

BRIAN SPEAKS

"Bodily I was there...
but my spirit was in the Garden of Eden."

In the three years since Brian began his talks, he has spoken to thousands of students in the Northern Virginia area. He never fails to captivate his audiences. About six months after he began with Bridget's assistance, everyone agreed he was ready to solo. These talks are Brian's lifeline. In so many other areas of his life, his disabilities limit his options, but as a public speaker delivering his message to teenagers, he is clearly gifted. His work has been recognized by The Washington Post (Levey), Reader's Digest (Mazie), local NBC television news, and several video producers, including Swedish Broadcasting in Washington, DC, and Channel Z Video Production in Arlington, Virginia.

The events related in the previous chapters reflect my viewpoint over the last eight years. Readers will be curious about Brian's perspective and recollections of these same events. For at least a year and a half after his accident, Brian's short-term memory (recording day to day events) was practically non- existent. Over the years, Brian has had many opportunities to read and comment on what I've written. In many cases, this reading has helped him put together some of the pieces of his journey, and in some instances he has made the text clearer by suggesting changes. Reading the early chapters sometimes renews intense feelings of grief over what he has lost.

As we considered ways to capture Brian's point of view for this book, we decided to ask him to re-read each chapter, beginning with Chapter 3. Then we asked survivor and friend Theresa Rankin (the circumstances of her brain injury are described in Chapter 6) to interview Brian. Those interviews were conducted in March 1993 without input from anyone else and were transcribed from audio tapes. The text that follows received only minimal editing.

Brian: I have read Chapter 3 to refresh that time period in my mind. Mom gave me this chapter yesterday and at one point I was crying so hard. It mentioned the pain that I caused my mother. And then at another point I was laughing!

Theresa: So when you read her text, you experience such a variety of feelings.

B: It was good to read it. I don't think I was doubtful at any time that it actually took place. Doubtful of my intentions, or my thoughts, according to her conclusions.

T: So when you read it now, you trust what it says.

B: So far, it does look pretty good. I will admit we haven't [yet] had too many altercations when my thinking came into play. I'm sure that will arise further in the book.

T: Can you talk about being at Mount Vernon Hospital (MVH)?

B: Most of the chapter is getting used to the place, meeting the people. I am barely able to hold my head up.

T: When you read your Mom's adjectives–courageous, interesting–is that part of what makes you laugh? You've never stopped being charming, interesting. Is that what helps you read the more difficult passages? Is that how you recall your experiences with the team at MVH?

B: Actually, I never thought in terms of a team. I felt more like a student with teachers. As with school, sometimes the teachers changed. People come, people go. Disheartening because the emotions that you attach to that person. . . I think it was all of Mount Vernon, everybody. I hold that time period at Mount Vernon–attach love to that time period. Everybody was there to help me get better.

T: And you rewarded their work, showed them the effort you put into every lesson. Do you think you surprised Dr. G. that you had that determination?

B: I don't want to think anybody can surprise Dr. G..

T: When you look at how they evaluated you in the beginning.

B: To this day I love to go back to Mount Vernon. I want to do that periodically. I want to go back and show myself off. The worst thing is everybody's changed. New people come in, old people leave. Chris Wade, my nurse, is no longer there. She works somewhere. It's very depressing. I loved the place called Mount Vernon Hospital, but the person who symbolizes MVH, Chris Wade, is no longer there. What do you do?

T: Chapter 3 describes the challenges that were there for you.

B: Not really, it describes the challenges when I first got there. In later chapters, it talks more about what I did at MVH. Then we will see the challenges that were there for me. This chapter is just moving into the place.

T: When you read about the time you spent in physical therapy, do you remember those things?

B: That's what's so funny. I was there, I should remember those times, but I can't. It's like I have told people I wasn't there. Bodily I was there, but my spirit was not there. That's very true, I think.

T: Where do you think your spirit was, Brian? In a safe spot, waiting?

B: Yes (weeping). My spirit was in the Garden of Eden.

T: Your Mom says that too –the person of who you are was coming into the real world again, coming out of a coma. Those are reflections of how strong your spirit was.

B: The <u>Washington Post</u> article about me –there was a sub-heading called "The Gradual Awakening in 5A-8" That's the one I stayed in.

T: Your Mom has written about some situations with Mary Beth Ireland.

B: She was my physical therapist, short and muscular.

T: So you remember the strength of people who were working with you.

B: I needed that strength, day in and day out. I would lose my balance, I would need her to catch me. If she didn't correct it, I would have hit the ground, but she stopped me from falling. Mary Beth, thank you so much.

T: Did you experience that same kind of steadiness with other people?

B: Well, no not really. Again, I'm looking mainly in a physical sense. In all the other therapies I couldn't physically touch the difference in myself. Everything was psychological and I couldn't measure how well psychologically I was doing. But you can measure how well you can walk.

T: You had that determination because you could see your progress.

B: It was the only place I could tell that I was doing anything, so that was the only place I tried to do a lot.

T: How about when you started speaking?

B: My ears were bad, so I sounded fine to myself. Also you can't judge your own voice. You're saying it, you know what you're saying, it may not sound like anything normal, but you know what you are saying. Why other people can't understand you, is beyond me. <u>You know what you're saying!</u>

T: Did it cause you a lot of anger when people couldn't understand what you were saying?

B: Yes, puzzled anger. Anger and frustration go hand in hand.

T: Did you find when your Mom or Dad came and prayed with you, did that relieve your frustration?

B: Well, I'm sure it did. My mother is a very spiritual person. I'm almost sorry that spirituality is not a big thing to me. I wish the spiritual part of my life was more important to me, so that I would be more on a level with my mother.

T: Isn't that spiritual when you talk of your spirit being in the Garden of Eden?

B: Yes, my spirit was coming back in this chapter and in the next.

T: Maybe your spirituality isn't less, just different. When you read about these prayers that you participated in, does that make you feel a connection?

B: Everything in a spiritual context, that's my mother. It's important to her. It is important what matters to me, but this is her book, so.

T: [We want to hear your] thoughts, your experiences, your connection to this material. Each part of the team was drawn into your strength.

B: My recollection of the chapter is there were only two or three parts of the team. Later there will be five or six parts of the team. Keeps getting bigger. This chapter I'm in elementary school, one teacher who gives you all the classes during a day. Then in junior high school, you go to different classes for different subjects, which is comparable to the next stage of rehab.

T: So when you read these words, you're seeing the advancements you're making, being able to think, walk. Do you have dreams about the past?

B: I'll tell you this, Theresa. Two maybe three times a day I will break down in tears for what I've lost, for what I could have been.

T: But are you also able to see how you've become stronger in so many areas.

B: Maybe psychologically stronger, but by no means would I trade that for a career with the airlines, flying jets, being married, a normal life. No way.

T: Were there certain people who helped you know more about what had happened?

B: Almost everybody there knew what I was going through. There was a time that they used to put me in a wheelchair. I always wanted to get away from that chair, I didn't realize that I needed that chair!

T: Were you able to see how other people reacted to you?

B: I didn't bother to look. I wanted to rant and rave about my problems and I didn't care about how anyone else dealt with it.

T: On Jan. 14, Dr. G. said, "We have a whole new chapter now." Were you aware of making progress?

B: Not at all, not at all. Honest to God, for the 13 months that I was there, I could see my advances in physical therapy, because that was physical. I could not see the mental changes that I made!

T: Were you more able as the months went by to understand what was going on around you?

B: When I was in MVH, just before I left there, I was self-transporting. That meant that I had to leave my room, and to come back, be where I was supposed to be to be picked up. That really made me feel like a big man. Put me in charge of myself. I felt like I was a very big kid! But that was only at the end of my time at MVH.

T: One of Dr. G's comments was, "When a head trauma survivor experiences too much stimuli, he shuts down or becomes agitated." Do you remember about that?

B: I think I did become agitated, but don't remember. Upset, yelling, angry. I don't know how I expressed that anger.

T: Your parents were concerned with the funding issues at MVH.

B: I didn't realize anything about that, I wanted to go home. But what home was, where it was, how it would be–none of those things mattered to me. I just wanted to go home. Then when I finally did get home, I found out how bad it was. I had changed, everybody in my house had changed.

T: While you were at MVH, what kind of emotion did you think you were experiencing then?

B: Why are you making me stay here? Why don't you take me home?

T: Your battle to become more physically able went on. When you read what it was that they were fighting for, does that make you more relaxed about why you were there?

B: It makes me shocked. I cannot believe, when I found out. My parents, my Mom, my Dad, both of them did so much for me. My God! How I would love to repay them. I wish all it would take is dollars and cents, because I would pay them and pay them well.

T: Do you think that each time you spoke, and each time you responded with laughter that you were repaying them, that you were coming back?

B: At that time I didn't realize, I didn't think Mom and Dad were doing anything. I wasn't grateful for anything, I hated them for making me stay there. I realize now, I know now. If I had been able to leave the hospital and come home, wetting my bed every night would not have gone over too well. Having to wear diapers, having to have my baby food ready in the morning would not have been good. A 20-year-old son who needs to eat baby food!

T: And when the fight to stay at Mount Vernon was won.

B: Medicaid didn't want to pay, Kaiser didn't want to pay and there was no way Mom and Dad could pay. I met this girl. Her family lives in a town house. They used to have a house like ours. Her parents sold their house so they could pay to put her through rehab. I cannot begin to fathom a system that lets that happen.

T: Chapter 3 ends on the reality that the battle really isn't over, that it's ongoing. Your individual progress is ongoing.

B: To this day, I don't think it's changing. It is definitely at a much slower rate than it was at that time. But it's still present.

T: It seems remarkable that your journey parallels your parents' journey in that they have ongoing goals, you have goals, and yet for each roadblock that comes in the way there's a psychological letdown.

B: My parents had goals and I had goals, but my parents' goals and my goals were not the same. My parents' goals were the goals that I would have in two or three months.

T: So they were working ahead of you.

B: Way far ahead of me sometimes. Most of my rehab I got before I was ready for it. A lot of it–Mom and Dad wanted me to get better fast–they didn't want me to go through the long process. I can't blame them– they're only human.

T: Part of what we were talking about was goals. Your parents' goals were months ahead of yours at times. Did you feel that your time at MVH in this beginning stage was an accomplishment?

B: It's so hard to say because the real Brian, the spiritual Brian was still in the Garden of Eden and not in me.I was trying to say that earlier, but I kept getting choked up. My body, my mind had to be... Could you imagine if I could remember all of it. Could you imagine being there when you say, "This is when I died –this is how I died. This is the way it felt–this is how it happened" (weeping). It's a blessing that my mind had left. I couldn't remember my girlfriend my sophomore year of college. Now that's when my memory loss was NOT a blessing. She was beautiful, red hair, gymnastics team (whistles). Really hot.

T: Thank you Brian, I think you've said what you want to say.

• • •

B: Chapter 4 really hurt me. It didn't explicitly say anything I didn't like, but it caused me to think and remember events and how twisted I was, how I hurt people because of what I did.

T: The sadness they experienced?

B: My mis-analyzing the case.

T: Chapter 4 talks about your day-to-day journey to recover.

B: It was really the first part of the chapter that bothered me. The second part was better–more talking about my accomplishments.

T: The opening line is, "No one could predict how long Brian's rehab would take."

B: I don't believe it will ever be done. That's the biggest difference between me and the people I live with at Cheshire [the group home in Arlington where Brian lived for one year]. They were born with their handicaps–they've grown up with their handicaps. They've never been on the outside. They're used to living in institutions or staying home. Maybe one or two have a job, but even then the people they meet are more consoling than making them work.

T: At the end of Chapter 3, "Brian showed his determination to live– to work at the essence of life, to speak, to eat, to remember."

B: I'm sorry, my mind is in the present, not yet thinking of myself three or four years ago. At that time I was coming out of my shell, coming out of coma –the door was opening up. It was kind of funny, those people that helped me at that time, like my parents. They were just ecstatic that Brian was awake. I was developing a pattern of "Everybody is so happy with me," so happy that I was doing anything. Now as I try to do more, I'm not good.

T: I think Chapter 4 is coming to understand– your family, the therapists, and for yourself that there would be periods of progress, coming up that mountain, and periods where you would level off, where you are not making as much gain.

B: I think I'm in one of the level off periods now.

T: You're at that plateau where you're kind of coasting.

B: Good analogy.

T: But for yourself, not only are you are so much different from before the injury, but you are different from others at Cheshire home because of your level of awareness, your level of understanding of all that can be done.

B: My level of acceptance, too. Having lived a normal life for 20 years, I know what I should be able to do.

T: Would you also agree that while life may not be the same, life holds an entirely new set of opportunities.

B: That's just a thought. I am so into focusing on what I've lost–I guess I'm still thinking of myself in terms of the pre-accident Brian. But if I put myself in post-accident Brian thinking–what with the talks to students, my minor attempt at a job at the Pentagon...

T: In Chapter 4, you were educating Chris Wade, just as she was educating you, you were educating her. You surprised them! You showed your determination to live, inspired the team at MVH to get past those points of anger and misunderstanding. When you read in this chapter, "your brain was still not quite awake, what do you imagine?"

B: *I can imagine what she means by "my brain was not fully awake yet," but I can't see when... it was awake to me, I can't see it. It's like all through rehab, not once did I see the progress I was making until I started to walk. That was the only physical thing I could see. All the cognitive things–sure, I'll play this stupid game with you. I don't think I'm doing anything different now than I did two weeks ago, but the progress was unbelievable. It was probably my bad memory, I don't know.*

T: The team were able to keep track of the measurements of progress.

B: *The team wrote down in the book to see my actions, reactions. Then they could look back and say, "You're so much better now." I didn't have a book. My memory was nowhere near a book. It was more like page after page–without the binding. There was no way I could look back.*

T: When I read about Chris Wade or someone writing in the book, congratulating you on your progress, I wondered if Brian had a book to write his thoughts, such as, "I'm so angry today at Chris."

B: *I think I had a memory book, but I didn't use it faithfully. It would have helped me quite a lot and it would help me now. Why I don't do it, I'll never know.*

T: I think I hear in the way you describe yourself, and the way you are determined to achieve goals, that you are problem solving now. And then you'll give yourself permission to let that goal happen.

B: *I don't know if I let it happen, but I want that goal to happen. I know there's more I need to accomplish.*

T: In Chapter 4 you refer to the therapists as teachers.

B: *I think they were teachers, not just the fact that they taught me something, but also in my attitude towards them. In my mind my therapists were in a different class than my nurse. My nurse was my "mom," my therapists were my teachers. Respect them both, but not the same. The different things that they helped me with, Chris with ADL's (Activities of Daily Living), Mary Beth with balance–physical things. At that early stage, I was just learning to talk and just learning to hold my head upright, instead of just letting it fall to the side, learning to look people in the eye.*

T: When you read about the effort you had to put into every movement, were you like a bear in hibernation, you know that image of the brain not quite awake yet?

B: I think the image of the brain not quite awake was more my own. I want to think I could have held my head up straight, but maybe I couldn't. I don't know why, but if I wanted to I think I could have. But I was more interested in going to sleep than working.

T: I think that's part of the mystery of the brain that this book is helping people understand. You wanted to walk, you wanted to hold your head up, but the other part of your brain was still asleep, was still in recovery. And your jaw being frozen in place, that took weeks.

B: It's going on, it's still going on, what happened today is an example. Quite often I find myself trying to eat too fast, and I know I need to take my time, but if I take the time I need, I go too slow.

T: I think it's valuable how you see a situation, for instance with your jaw, how what was happening in Chapter 4 relates to the present, how you've gained full command of your voice.

B: You are in a seat that I never sit in, you're hearing me–how do I sound to you–do I sound like another adult?

T: Yes, I hear an adult voice that's measured by serious thought and that what you're saying is of importance and is from the heart and that it's going to be worth my listening to.

B: When you said "from the heart" that made me think about a line from a Louis L'Amour book that I read. "He was a good man–he smiled from the heart–and a lady can always love a man who smiles from the heart."

T: Brian, in the year and a half that I've been back, I see progress in your voice. It's not too high, it's not too low. It carries the sound of the words you're saying. What these conversations show is that you were fully present, and on the days when your brain wasn't going to let you participate, you were asleep!

B: Unhunh.

T: You were on a sabbatical and your brain was developing energy.

B: It's funny. Maybe I'm just trying to get it awake in that chapter. Now I'm trying to get it to fly. Maybe that's it. That could be the big step.

T: Some concern was expressed in this chapter about your ability to judge how far you could walk or what you could do. I think some passages show that your judgment was very good. Your mother describes when they built a playpen of plywood in order to give you as much freedom as possible. Then she says, "That arrangement was never acceptable to him." Your judgment was that this isn't the best way for me to get back into action, so they gave you the tiered arrangement.

B: I can remember that, the tiers of mattresses. I can remember having two mattresses, one mattress, then the floor (laughs).

T: Why does that make you laugh?

B: Because I just thought of one time when I was lying in the upper bed, and I had to go to the bathroom while I was asleep. So I just rolled over onto the next mattress and slept there!

T: Your decision-making was pretty prompt. I don't want to stay here! I think that's a certain kind of accommodation–the objective is to be sleeping comfortably and you found the next best place. Another example when Dr. G. recommended a helmet and your parents purchased a bicycle helmet, but you preferred the batter's helmet and you were willing to wear that.

B: More like the old Brian. My memory tells me I hated helmets, baseball helmets were fine, but other helmets were–you see epileptics wearing helmets. They have a seizure, they may fall down, so they have to wear a helmet to protect their head. I don't have seizures, but I do fall down. Maybe I should wear a helmet.

T: And was that your thinking process–you didn't think you and your body were out of control so you didn't want to wear a helmet? But there was a level of acknowledging that the batter's helmet was OK.

B: And then with my bad memory, later in the day I couldn't remember that I'd fallen down and hurt myself. I couldn't remember that, so when they said, "Brian, you have to wear your helmet; you fell down today," I would say, "I never did that!"

T: The day-to-day living at MVH was about accepting assistance.

B: It was about accepting my shortcomings, learning what they were. I will find out even better through more rehab, but at that time I was just barely awake and not functioning fully.

T: So in Chris's entries in the book, she speaks of the ADL's, the stepping stones for daily living, and you have them down pat now. Chapter 4 is also about your re-emerging and being more aware that you were in a hospital and in some ways being kept there, yet the part of your mind that did the thinking...

B: That's the hardest thing. The thinking part of my brain was injured, but the thinking part of my brain is asking why was I there and the thinking part is coming up with answers, but it is the thinking part that is injured. So those answers are no good. But the physical part of my brain follows what the thinking part tells it to do.

T: In the second part of the chapter, you can see that your brain was giving you so many mixed signals. You began walking and began to express your desire to come home, yet everything around shows that you are in the most supportive place. But the thinking part of your brain said, "I don't need to be here."

B: That's the injured part and that "I don't need to be here" idea was not correct.

T: One thing that is amazing is the special sense of humor that you have. When someone would say, "Brian, do you know who this is?" And you would say, "Of course," and come up with a really funny line. Your sense of humor was a lifesaver for everyone involved.

B: It was my way of coping with a bad memory, to make light of forgetting. But you can't always do that in the outside world, not today's world.

T: There are ongoing challenges. You were in a training program, as if to be a Navy Seal, facing the physical, cognitive, and emotional demands to see how much progress you can make. And it goes on for an entire year. This chapter is about the beginning of a lifetime. Do you remember when Dr. Patrick became part of the team?

B: Only in BRIDGE do I remember Dr. Patrick. I can't remember him from MVH. My brain became more awake and more able to remember at that point.

T: You were also using the tools that you were learning. Is that what your "book" was about.

B: My book was to write down the events of that day–what therapies there were and what I did, just so I could refer back to them and say, "Wow, look at this–that is two steps beyond that."

T: So you did have a sense of the measurement.

B: If I wrote things down, I would have, but I didn't.

T: Not consistently.

B: If I did consistently, I lost it. That may be why I don't record things any more. I don't know what it is–there is a mysterious goblin that comes in and steals my things. It's not me that loses them. The mysterious goblin wants to mess up my life.

T: So that is the enemy that you are fighting.

B: That is incorrect, but that's what the injured mind is telling me.

T: Your Mom identifies that the testing they did showed that your memory was very fragmented, you couldn't hold on to the sequence of anything.

B: I couldn't remember at 10:00 what I did at 9:00. Now I can remember what I did at 9:00 at 12:00, but at 2:00 I might not be able to do that. And if I learned back at the beginning to write things down, I would remember what I did, but I didn't.

T: Your Mom writes that the process was elusive and complex; she describes what she has seen you go through, the memory that is hot and cold. She identifies that you had a conspiracy theory about why you were kept at the hospital. Does that fit in with your understanding now—your brain was receiving mixed messages?

B: Those are the things that hurt me about this chapter. It's those things I did that hurt others. I didn't mean for them to hurt others, but they did.

T: I think it's acknowledged that your Mom does understand. She decided to stop visiting for a while to protect herself. I think she understood what was taking place.

B: I believe at that time when Mom stayed away for a week, I remember saying to Dad, "I haven't seen mother for a long time," not realizing that every time I saw her I gave her a hard time about something, not realizing that—just realizing that I hadn't seen her in a long time.

T: Part of what I see here is the partnership of your parents, coming to the team meetings, to talk about progress and concerns and areas of hurt that were taking place for them and for you in the struggle to come forward. Your Dad said to you, "You are a winner," and that you needed to believe in that.

B: I remember that, "Brian, you are a winner."

T: That's the power of an affirmation. Your father was speaking from the heart, believing in that. And when Scott came to see you, perhaps this was the first time you could see the bigger picture. Remember the festival, the helicopter, the ambulance: the two of you talked about that and you realized that you had been rescued.

B: Medevac. I look at people who do that with respect and reverence. Even though it happened to me, I still have trouble believing it.

T: Scott was helping you see your reality when you saw that helicopter—helping you to move on and stop struggling with why you were at MVH.

B: To see the big picture, see what happened to me.

T: You were also aware of people who were your champions. You talked about therapy sessions, working on the keyboard, you said, "I like the audience, sort of a cheering section." Did that give you energy to have people cheering?

B: I'm a natural-born showoff!

• • •

T: When you read about coming home in Chapter 5, did you relive some of that time?

B: It's funny, it's so much. At no point in this chapter was I reduced to tears. Quite often in the other chapters, I would read about something I felt strongly about and those feelings would come back to me. But there was none of that in Chapter 5. Maybe I'm just accepting it easier.

T: Do you think that was a big part of your emotional growth, accepting day-to-day events?

B: I hope so, that makes me sound pretty good.

T: I sense that your self-esteem is much stronger, that your self-awareness is much more.

B: Being able to handle talking about myself.

T: It's a very big step. In this chapter, your mother describes some of your interaction with Scott. You're standing in the kitchen and are going to move from one spot to the next. Scott stood there and didn't quite know what to do, to help or to wait. When you read that, do you see?

B: It seemed faintly familiar. I must be wrong, but I would hope that such a dramatic instance would be better placed in my memory, but obviously it wasn't. I don't know, it's kind of scary that I would –that I couldn't even protect myself.

T: Do you think it scared your family when you first came home; your family was afraid for you?

B: At that time I was still more of a newborn baby than a 20 year old, and they were out to protect me more. My other siblings must have felt ripped off. I shouldn't say my other siblings, I should say my younger siblings.

T: Because so much attention was paid to your every movement?

B: At that young age, I guess they needed attention. Then having an older brother who needs so much. I think they still feel some anxiety, some anger towards me.

T: Do you think it's just some ongoing emotions that are being worked on?

B: They're mad at me for having this accident and messing up their lives.

T: Do you think that's ongoing?

B: It will be until they get old enough to accept it as a bad happening. My older brother gets along with me fine, but he is older and can accept it. The younger ones are still...

T: Still very young.

B: Still very young. I guess the worst part is Eric. I mean he was a freshman when I had my accident. He's about as physical as I was, even more so; I used to play football with him, play basket ball, wrestle, just physical things. It hurts him that I can't do those things any more. It hurts him that I had the accident. It hurts me that I had the accident. I'm sorry, I'm focusing on myself.

T: No, I think you're in focus, you're talking about how the family changed because of this tremendous loss. You were still Brian, but so much had been lost. You're identifying that Eric lost a big brother that he had a very strong and physical relationship with, camaraderie. To have that changed so dramatically has been hard for both of you.

B: I wish sometimes I had the key to turn back time (weeping).

T: You're dealing with some very deep issues for the whole family, but you're identifying that emotion for all kinds of people. It's not just who you are in the family, it's how the whole family is still changing.

B: They're having to relearn–they were just learning who their big brother was, when all of a sudden he changed.

T: Then you came home in January 1987; you came home and there was danger in everything, that you might fall...

B: I was so much like a little kid, so much. Every little thing, Brian could hurt himself. I was unable to protect myself. It talks about me hitting my head and it was just symbolic. I didn't know I was falling backwards until my head hit the ground. With my mixed up senses I really didn't feel the knock on the head, just felt the results (whirring noises). Wow, I did hit my head!

T: The beginning of this chapter talks about your coming home from the hospital where all of your needs were taken care of. An opportunity for you to become your own person again, cook your meals, do your laundry.

B: Coming home to the house that I lived in for 20 years and nothing looks the same. Granted with time everything changes, but my house is never going to change that much. Maybe it was just my bad memory, partly that I've changed, partly that my viewpoint changed. I mean I was no longer standing, I was sitting in a wheelchair. Everybody's attitude toward me had changed.

T: Are you aware of how attitudes changed in this chapter; how they had to let you take risks.

B: I take risks, but I don't really see them as risks. At that time, they were just things to be done. I might hurt myself, so what! It might make me better. Anything that will make me better, I've got to do.

T: Were you relearning a lot of new rules?

B: I was learning about how a head injury is like being reborn, you really learn all about yourself all over again. I used to wear Attends right after my accident; then I was in a wheelchair for a while. A

*wheelchair is a self-propelled stroller. It's like growing up–I'm prob-
ably 15 years old now mentally, maybe older than that. But the aging
process goes so much faster the second time than the first time, when it
took me 20 years to get to where I am, and it's taken me eight years to
get back to where I was!*

T: How do you experience that aging that is going on?

*B: It's just the difference in you, from age 20 to 25, I mean five years,
yes. A little bit older looking, but what does it do to you as a person; it
changes you. That's the aging process.*

T: Who do you talk with when you want to talk about different issues?

*B: Scott, he's my "big brother." He's been there, he knows. He said to
me one time, "Any time you have weird thoughts, you think someone did
something; before you act, call me, tell me and I'll tell you if it really
happened or not." "How will you know?" "I'll know–I may call you
back later that day, but I will know."*

T: So you have a partnership, an agreement, with Scott.

*B: The two of us used to share this room, can you imagine Scott and I
in this room. At that time I was 9 months and he was three years, a little
bit smaller than we are now. Scott's about 6 foot 2, but he weighs less
than I do. Everyone here weighs less than I do.*

T: That partnership with Scott has been very valuable. How about your
ability to talk to your mother?

*B: Inasmuch as I change. Over the years as I change, over the years as
she changes, our ability to get along changes.*

T: In 1987, that was really your starting point again.

*B: It was a big step for me [coming home from the hospital]. I only saw
it as "I'm out, I'm free." But the people here couldn't see that. For
instance my sister used to have the downstairs room all to herself,
coming from that big room to taking this small room. It's like I'm so
sorry I made you do that–I didn't realize that.*

T: Did you talk with the members of your family about these things?

*B: I didn't see these things, didn't see them till I was reading this chapter
now! It's like my vision inward is not that good. By hearing someone
else's idea of what has happened, I get a biased idea. It's their own idea
of what happened, what they feel happened.*

T: Is Scott the one that helps you find the balance? Someone else has
their viewpoint, how do you find a middle ground? Other people in your
family have a bias. Scott seems to have a good understanding; is he the
one who helps you stay on balance?

B: He's the one who helps me stay in line. He keeps me going upward and not crooked, to the side. He kicks me in the butt and says, "Straighten out, kid!"

T: And what is it he's helping you straighten out?

B: Making me see that I have not gone straight. You can tell me but that's not making me see, making me see. I can't tell you exactly what it is.

T: Is it about a way of understanding an argument, a talk.

B: How others feel about it, how they see it.

T: Does that take away some of the anger, defensiveness that you may have?

B: Sometimes when they tell me how they saw it, it reminds me of what I felt when I was living it, and then I get angry all over again.

T: A lot of that feeling comes from deep inside–in the heart.

B: Here (touching chest).

T: When you went through the BRIDGE program, were some of those things dealt with there, or was BRIDGE just daily living?

B: Well, there were a lot of cognitive things, thinking or reasoning things, but I think I was still focusing mainly in the physical sense so if it wasn't physical therapy, I didn't want to do it.

T: That's right, you wanted to walk.

B: I finally learned to do it at the end of Chapter 5, down at Woodrow Wilson. You know it's really funny, I was in this class called CCES, and they were going to train me for a job and they gave me a vocational evaluation testing. I failed vocational evaluation, mainly because I was still in a wheelchair at that time. I didn't want vocational evaluation, I wanted to walk. You know, don't bother giving me a job, get me on my feet and then I'll get a job! Big problem is now I'm on my feet and I've got a helluva job. $30 for two weeks work! [Brian works on bulk mailing at Fairfax Opportunities Unlimited, a sheltered workshop for people with disabilities.]

T: Is it true though that for each step you take, it's another part of the puzzle?

B: There's always been another hurdle to jump over; something unexpected has come up, always.

T: Part of what's talked about in this chapter is that strong goal to walk, and another strong goal was to be able to drive.

B: I'm sure it was a strong urge. I did not realize my own handicap. You know I can remember so well that day I took Sheri's car. I can remember driving around–I can remember turning onto a street and seeing a cop ahead of me with a car pulled over. I mean if the cop saw me he would have come after me! I just wanted to get away. Again, just a kid, still a little kid. Mom and Dad shouldn't have worried. I didn't have a prayer in passing the eye test for driving.

T: That was a frightening moment for your mother that day.

B: The weirdness of being behind the wheel again...

T: Had you been planning that for a long time?

B: Not planning it–wanting it, but I didn't give it a second thought, spontaneity. That's also what got me behind the wheel. Nobody was home. Here are the keys, I'm gone, I'll be back before Mom gets home, no problem. Oh God (sigh).

T: And do you remember what happened when your Mom got home?

B: I came up the street and saw Mom's car in the driveway. Oh God I'm late; Mom's early. Oh no–I pulled in. Mom started to yell at me and I rolled the windows back up. When you calm down, I'll come in. I fell asleep. It was good for me; I needed it as much as she did.

T: You wrote when you described going for that drive, "I felt free like a bird must feel when it flies, but puzzled by my erratic driving." Was that a significant experience?

[Here Brian gestured to his collection of L"Amour books–his favorite author since high school.]

B: See all those books, I've read every single one of them. I like to read, maybe I'm bored quite a bit and I like to read, but because I read a lot, my vocabulary is very good.

T: Do you find freedom in reading?

B: That's a difficult question. I never thought about it–freedom in reading.

T: You enjoy Louis L'Amour.

B: I must escape, I must jump into the character and live the parts, I don't know.

T: Do you find freedom with your family?

B: I don't know.

T: Do you find support and encouragement for your dreams and ideas?

B: Yes, I guess I do. Let's get back to the book.

T: But that's what this chapter is about, Brian! Chapter 5 is about your coming home and rebuilding your relationship with your family, so that when they gave you help, you felt that support. You stayed at BRIDGE for four sessions–then you were accepted at Woodrow Wilson?

B: What happened was that they gave me vocational evaluation and I was still in a wheelchair. I didn't want vocational evaluation, I wanted to walk, so I failed vocational evaluation on purpose because I wanted to learn to walk! I'm walking, I've got no job though. Am I happy, no. But if I had a job but was not walking, would I be happy? Probably not!

T: This last part of Chapter 5 talks about exploring, going to Pennsylvania, going to Texas.

B: Looking for someplace for me to live? When I first read that, I wondered whatever happened to Pittsburgh? I am a warm weather nut, California would be terrific.

T: Part of what your parents discovered was that the cost was too high.

B: Not only was the cost too high, but I know now I would never put up with Mom and Dad paying for it. I had the accident, they shouldn't have to suffer any more.

T: Part of what your parents were looking at was whether DRS [Department of Rehabilitative Services] could cover the costs. And DRS just couldn't do it, could they? So the family agreed that life would be taken one day at a time. You also discovered the friends that you had in Springfield.

B: Mr. Bounds used to come and get me every morning without fail, pick me up, take me up to the high school. They would leave the gates open, he would drive across the field and park beside the running track, then he would walk around the car, help me out and walk with me around the track. Wow! And I'm only a neighbor kid and he did that for me. I can understand doing it for your own kid, but for a neighbor.

T: It was a tremendous gift.

• • •

T: Maybe we should start with the best part of Chapter 6. You found your voice. Your mother came to the realization that she had to let go of you more, to let you become an independent person.

B: It made me feel good when she first gave me that "Letting Go" poem. She gave it to me when I went away to college, so when she gave it to me the second time, I figured I must be at the same level. All right!

T: You were celebrating the gains you made. A lot of what's talked about is the struggle that goes on for the family in becoming more aware of what your life will become and trying to find resources. Your mother says it was a very difficult time. Where would the resources be to take you into independent living? She says you began to realize how hard your parents worked as advocates on your behalf.

B: I already see how hard they fought for me, but I am afraid that the amount I think they fought for me is a pittance to what they really fought for me, to get me to where I am. Do you remember the story of the mother killing her son and then herself? So, but it's understandable too, almost understandable. I don't know—it hurts that that stuff happens.

T: Is it hurting because it seems that people run out of hope?

B: It hurts because they figured there was no hope. That death would be better.

T: In going to the Head Injury Association support group meetings, did you find a lot of hope there from other survivors?

B: If I still had my pocket talker or some good way to hear what's happening in a small group, it would be good. But as it is I'm good in a one-on-one, but you get two or three people and I just can't follow–I can't understand–if he's talking to you, I can't hear him. I don't know what's being said, so for fear of sounding off-the-wall, I don't say anything.

T: So your best interaction is one-on-one, for instance talking with Melissa about searching for a job.

B: It's easier for me to talk to a group of students because I'm more or less talking to a group and then when they ask questions at the end, one of them comes up front and stands next to me and repeats the questions.

T: Was that a valuable lesson to learn about your hearing ability and about how to stay in communication?

B: It was easy. When I said, "Are there any questions?" and the first person raised his hand, I pointed to him and, "Mumble, mumble, mumble." What? "Mumble, mumble." It's not working! Then I asked for someone to come up and help me!

T: That's a very valuable skill, knowing how to ask for help, knowing how to identify what you need.

B: In a way, it's harmful to ask for help.

T: In what way?

B: I don't even attempt to do it myself, I ask before I even attempt. It's like I'm in a department store and instead of finding the men's department on my own, I'll ask and then tomorrow when I come back, I'll ask. And then the next day I'll ask again. They kind of get tired of constantly telling me. I told you once, twice, don't you know? I didn't write it down. I'm sorry, but that's what I should have done. I really have to start writing things down. Why don't I do that? I carry a calendar. Why don't I write things down? Do you write things down?

T: Yes.

B: What do you write down?

T: Almost everything. I write directions to where I'm going, a reminder of how to use the map. I have notes here for our interview, so I would have a structure, the key points. I write down all my appointments. I use my calendar and my log for almost everything so that I can stay connected and can learn.

B: I don't stay connected, I ask. That's where asking is harmful, it's harmful to my independence. Also it makes people feel sorry for me, because I'm always asking and they feel, "We have to help that kid. He doesn't know anything, so we've got to help him."

T: And so how are you working to change that?

B: I'm just beginning to realize it.

T: Very good.

B: I don't know how I'm going to change it. Obviously write things down. I have pockets. I carry my calendar; I've got paper. I don't always have a pen. I guess I don't often get things that I have to remember. Maybe it's not knowing what I need to remember. Maybe it's not just pull out the calendar and write it down. It's pull out the calendar, zip, open it up to the right page. Oh no, I forgot the pen. Zip.

T: All the steps involved.

B: Takes too long, still independence is worth the interruptions. Independence is the biggest four letter word I've ever heard.

T: I think Chapter 6 identifies how you found your voice, your connection to the community. When you began to work with Rhonda Woodward at DRS, that's when doors began opening; that's how you found a job.

B: Speaking of a job, that Pentagon job, I chastise myself. I guess I just didn't see the reality of it all, didn't understand that yelling at that boss was going to get me not to work at the Pentagon any more! I wore nice shirts, ties, learned how to tie a tie, wear dress shoes, dress pants, socks.

T: Perhaps we can set the stage better by acknowledging that the support system wasn't yet in place, that your rehab counselor, the job coach, and the supervisor herself didn't have an awareness yet.

B: It hurts me to be so dependent, only because I'm scrabbling for my independence, to put myself in a position where I need to be dependent. Maybe right now, not writing things down I make myself dependent.

T: Do you think that was one of the steps that brought about the end of the Pentagon job? You weren't writing things down.

B: I thought I always did. I thought every file I gave out I recorded, but I wasn't the only one that could go into the files. Maybe it was somebody else. I don't know. But it doesn't matter, I still got blamed.

T: Part of what was learned from that situation was that more cooperation needed to be put in place, with the supervisor being more educated, your job coach more familiar with developing strategies, with you yourself being an equal in that partnership.

B: We all needed to work together.

T: What you were experiencing at that job was taking more control of your own progress. Was that a real exciting experience for you?

B: It really was, a dynamic place. Better yet, I met a young lady there. I went the wrong way to the cafeteria one day and I walked by her and after about 10 steps, I stopped. Good God, that girl was gorgeous. I retraced my steps. The next day I went the same way and I didn't see her. Never did see her again.

T: A big place to work.

B: Very big. I forget what the exact number of people that work there, but it's huge.

T: Big place to start. Part of what your Mom talked about in this chapter was your concern that people were taking things from you.

B: Me and my imagination, it's a bad memory that tells me that I put something here, and actually I put it there. Since I think I put it there, and it's not there, I think somebody stole it and I'm going to go and raise hell, instead of looking around.

T: Is that still a big issue for you?

B: I hope it's not (laughs). I hope it's not.

T: One of the best parts of this chapter is your meeting Bridget Wyrick.

B: Oh, starting those talks. Ahhhh (satisfied sigh). They've really been the strongest, biggest part of my life, doing those talks. I hope you can imagine, when I do those talks, I feel like a father, like I'm putting my arm around my kid saying "Son, daughter, I screwed up. Here's how. Don't let it happen to you." That's the way I feel. It's pretty nice. At last count, there were 4,000 kids that have heard my talk.

T: That's a remarkable number.

B: That's pretty good. That's pretty good.

T: I was impressed with your mother saying that the first time she heard you speak, she felt such a joy in hearing you tell your story, that you were like a valedictorian.

B: That is at the survivor panel. I just got to the part in Chapter 6 where Tom Stumm was telling his story.

T: How did that story affect you?

B: That's what really made me feel that I need to write things down. Tom has learned–I think it's about time that I learned. It's taken me a long time–I don't know why it's taken so long.

T: We all have a different amount of acceptance and willingness. Do you know Tom very well?

B: Because of my hearing problems, I can't really understand him when he talks, so we can't really converse, but I know who Tom is and Tom

knows who Brian is. Of course he's probably got it written down.
T: That's right, he most likely has it in his address book. I think one of the themes I see throughout the book is that with each step of progress you are gaining more ability. First in developing this speech for the survivors panel and then going to the high schools with Bridget. That is really a whole new life for you.
B: The survivors panel speech goes almost parallel to my speech that I give to high schools.
T: And that speech talks about living in the real world.
B: At the end it does. The high school speech talks about living in the real world.
T: Have you ever found any of the high school presentations to be challenging. Or are all the students just surprised?
B: I've been surprised at the questions they ask. One of the young adults asked me, "Why do you want to do this?" Wow, what an indepth question. Then on the other hand, one of the kids said, "How old are you?" You get a wide range of questions.
T: And how did you answer that question?
B: That was easy. I want to do these talks because I messed up my life by not wearing my seatbelt. I don't want to see others mess up their life by not wearing a seatbelt. One is too many.
T: If you could get a job doing that...
B: God, I would love it! I would love it. Good heavens. This is my wildest dream, being able to have an 800 number, FOR TALK, and then have any school, any organization, in the whole United States, Alaska and Hawaii included, be able to call me up. We'd like Brian Rife to come on such and such date–transportation all paid for. Then I would get on an airplane and fly to Alaska. Oh God, I would love it! I would really rise to the occasion. Yes ma'am, it would make me feel very good. I have a message for the kids. I just need them to hear me.
T: I've heard you speak, Brian, and I know that you can do it far better than anyone else. Then I think of how when you were at Woodrow Wilson in 1989 and how they listed you as vocationally untrainable!
B: Let me explain to you why they came up with that. They have something called vocational evaluation. They gave that to me and I failed it. I was in a wheelchair. I wanted to get out of that chair more than I wanted to work. Big problem is that now I'm out of that chair, but I don't have any job and I'm not happy.
T: But they were looking at that wheelchair and testing you to see if maybe you could do accounting or bookkeeping, or to be a draftsman.

B: You're right, but you see the baseball helmet, see the trophies, I am a very physical person. I used to have a BB gun. I have a bowling ball. I just can't imagine living the rest of my life from a wheelchair. True, using canes is a little bit better than a wheelchair, not quite as good as walking. Give me time; that's all I say, give me time.

T: But Woodrow Wilson was testing you in a very limited area. So here you are in 1993 and you have proven your vocational skill as a speaker, as an educator, as an advocate for young people to be aware of safety issues.

B: Also in the fall of 1992 I started a job. It's been almost a year and I'm learning to mind my manners. But it's too late, I've already lost that Pentagon job.

T: But you're always working on your skills, a new level of social interaction and social ability.

B: I am a social person. I love to be friendly to everybody; I don't like to make enemies. Occasionally I do, but occasionally everybody does.

T: Brian, when you're working on big issues, do you have an outside counselor who can help you develop strategies?

B: I have a neuropsychologist, his name is Dr. Wires. Then Marianne Talbot of Head Injury Services Partnership, then Rhonda Woodward of DRS. Too many people in my head.

T: And are they effective advocates?

B: DRS is a good advocate, and Marianne is a good advocate. Dr. Wires is good to kick me in the butt and make me advocate for myself.

T: He likes to challenge you. Sounds like a good support system. What are your goals now, Brian?

B: A paying job, someplace to go every day that pays a decent hourly wage. The job I have now pays a piece wage and I only make $30 for two weeks. It's not very good money.

T: Hard to be independent when income is limited.

B: That's why I'm so angry that I lost the Pentagon job. I used to bring home $350 for two weeks. That is very good money.

T: Do you see yourself having gained ground with your self esteem?

B: That's the blessing of a bad memory. My mind does not stay on what I've lost, tends to forget that; be it good, be it bad, but it forgets it.

T: So you live in the present, right here, right now.

B: What I've lost is water under the bridge, already gone by and what I will be I don't know. It should be what I'm aiming for, what I'm working for. That's where Dr. Wires comes in, to kick me in the butt, make me do things, very good head shrink.

T: What would you like to see happen with this book, a part 2– part 3?

B: I don't know but I think maybe a book by me–Brian Rife does his own story (laughs) maybe it's My Book About Me. I have My Book About Me. I made that book when I was about 4 years old– pictures, dot to dot, color in the square, big lettering. Ohh, it's funny.

T: Do you have a sense of hope, a sense of opportunity?

B: If I didn't have a sense of hope, I wouldn't have anything.

T: And is that sense of hope built around a lot of people?

B: About my situation, about my lack of a good paying job, about doing talks for a living. That's something I would really love.

.8.

EPILOGUE

... the power of the world always works in circles..
even the seasons form a great circle in their changing, and always come
back again to where they were.

–Black Elk, Oglala Sioux

People who know only a little of our story will often ask me, "How is Brian now?" The answer is never simple. If I consider the young man of 20 who headed for the beach in July of 1985, look at his high school graduation picture, or see in my youngest son Dan the likeness of Brian 10 years ago, I can drift into grieving, and sometimes I allow myself that moment. But if I consider that in October of 1985 Brian was given almost no chance to regain *any* higher brain function, his current abilities are an extraordinary achievement, even miraculous!

LOOKING BACK

I have earned no advance degrees, received no professional training, and have not participated in any scientific rehabilitation research programs. I have only my PhE (Parent having Experience) and the benefit of a number of recent newspaper and journal articles written on rehabilitation. Looking back on the last eight years, I can see many places where things might have been done differently–in the Maryland trauma center, at Mount Vernon Hospital, in the vocational guidance Brian has been given, and in steps toward his re-integration in the community.

In the very beginning, when we were in shock trauma, professionals who spoke with us would have been wise to avoid predictions. They gave us the false impression they knew a lot more than we did. Neurosurgeons and others who work in trauma care must find time to talk to brain injury survivors 5, 10, 15 years after their injuries, and open dialogue with staff in rehabilitation centers, community re-entry programs, and nursing homes to broaden their viewpoint. I have no reason to believe that the art of prognosis in cases of traumatic brain injury has progressed very far in the last eight years.

After an injury like Brian's the course of events is extremely volatile and unpredictable. All the systems of mind and body are in chaos. The risks of secondary infections are very high and every precaution must be taken to guard the fragile recovery process. It has always seemed to us that Brian's meningitis could have been prevented, if the planned surgery to repair the tear in his cerebrospinal membrane had been accomplished more quickly. Even the ordinary precaution of a sterile environment seemed lacking in the chaotic atmosphere at shock-trauma in Baltimore. Professionals and family members responsible for decisionmaking at that early stage must recognize the extreme peril of any delays in treatment. Although it is impossible to determine which of Brian's disabilities were caused by the original injury and which were caused by the meningitis, clearly the meningitis was an additional devastating blow in that fragile early period.

We don't know the cause of Brian's hearing loss, a significant factor in his everyday challenges, but at least one doctor who is intimately familiar with his case history speculated it could have been caused by the powerful antibiotics used to arrest the raging spinal meningitis infection. We have no idea if alternative treatments were considered.

All families who have a relative in trauma as a result of a brain injury should immediately be given information about support groups, such as the National Head Injury Foundation sponsors. Not everyone will choose to follow up with this contact, but everyone deserves to receive the information. We have heard repeatedly of social workers who decide that a family is "not ready." This judgment cannot be made by anyone other than family members themselves.

No reliable statistics are available, but I am certain that among the people cared for in nursing homes nationwide are those (some very young) who sustained a brain injury and were placed there prematurely, when additional stimulation and therapy in those early months could have made a difference. Considering how hard we had to fight for funding and continued therapy when Brian's future hung in the balance, it is easy to imagine how many people have neither the energy nor the knowledge to stand up to insensitive systems. Using sophisticated medical technology to save a life, and then consigning that person prematurely to maintenance care is a horrendous injustice.

What do families need? Families need support and plenty of encouragement to talk about feelings, not just during the initial trauma, but for the long haul. Families need a spiritual base, a faith to carry them through an experience like ours. I like the phrase, "pray as if everything depended on God, and act as if everything depended on me." But faith is only part of the story. Rehabilitation costs money, a lot of money. Families must not leave decisions only to those who are tasked with cost control. To make matters more complicated, families can also be manipulated into thinking the most costly programs are the best. My own advice would be to look for rehabilitation that demonstrates imagination and a willingness to interact fully with other factors in the injured person's life–friends, family, co-workers.

There is growing evidence that rehabilitation can be done, and done well, for considerably less than Brian's 13-month inpatient rehabilitation at Mount Vernon Hospital. Was that 13 months of care (60 days funded by Kaiser-Permanente and the remainder by Virginia Medicaid), a good investment? There is no easy answer to that question, but ironically health maintenance organizations (HMOs) like Kaiser-Permanente (that seemed so ill-equipped to manage Brian's care eight years ago) may have an excellent opportunity to contribute to the development of newer models of care that combine client-centered rehabilitation and cost effectiveness. However, when I recently contacted the Chief Executive Officer of Kaiser-Permanente in California, requesting a commitment to improved services for people with head injury in Kaiser's many centers across the country, I received no reply. In the country's current debate about healthcare delivery and costs, these issues must be addressed.

Perhaps my contribution to the debate is to examine in some detail how Brian's rehabilitation "might" have been done better and more cost effectively. From the time of his injury in July of 1985 till June 1986, Brian certainly required complete inpatient care, and we have a sense of gratitude for all of the dedicated professionals who worked with him in three hospitals, especially Mount Vernon Hospital. But in the summer of 1986, Brian began to be more aware, asking for contact with the outside world, struggling mightily to make sense out of what was happening to him. The decision not to allow this contact until much later had more to do with the inflexibility of Medicaid rules and the shortcomings of a medical model of rehabilitation than with Brian's personal needs. A client-centered system of delivery would have been more sensitive to his wishes, even when his self assessment was very poor and his wishes seemed absurd.

An example of this principle came to my attention recently when

I had an opportunity to visit a rehabilitation facility in California. This facility in Vallejo, the only one of its kind operated by Kaiser-Permanente, works with people recovering from stroke, spinal cord injury and brain injury. Because some unique needs arise during the course of recovery from a brain injury, Vallejo has a contract with Neurocare in Davis where 24 hour one-on-one attention is provided during the more volatile stages. According to one of the neuro-psychologists at Vallejo, "One brain injury survivor wanted to run across the field, so the therapist [at Neurocare] ran alongside him!" This man, who had entered the agitated stage on the Rancho scale, was obviously much more mobile than Brian at that stage.

What if, in Brian's case, when he wanted to drive, someone sat beside him in a vehicle with dual controls and let him drive! Or when he wanted to come home, what if the system had enough flexibility to provide therapy and nursing in the home setting temporarily. It seems most likely that Brian would have gained a clearer picture of his actual situation, and then been able to work more consciously with rehabilitation plans. No doubt more real-life experiences would have been painful for him, but what right do we (parents or professionals) have to deny a person access to his life? Unnecessary dependency is created and the outcome is altered when rehabilitation is managed with little concern for the injured person's perception of reality.

The reasons why none of this could be done are mostly systemic. Virginia Medicaid rules state that if anyone is able to stay at home overnight, that person can be discharged from the hospital and the funding is stopped. The business aspect of the large inpatient rehabilitation hospitals dictates that they keep their "beds" as full as possible, a factor that often is not in the best direct interest of the person being rehabilitated. Another factor in Brian's case was the absence of a transitional living center affiliated with Mount Vernon Hospital. When this type of facility is available, movement out of the inpatient setting (and the attendant cost saving) is accomplished more quickly.

Vocational training and placement programs too, seem generally unable to respond to creative insight or coordinate effectively with other factors taking place in the person's life. Surprisingly, Brian's vocational counselors have never seen the employment potential in his prevention talks to students. One counselor even said to him, "Brian, do you want to do talks, or do you want to work?" implying that he had to make an absolute choice between what he loves–what truly serves the community–and unimaginative, low-paying work!

As Brian's parents, we too made errors in judgment. Having learned early in the process that we had to fight for what was needed, we probably pushed too hard for Brian's entry into some programs. As Brian said, "Most of my rehab I got before I was ready for it." I can see where we took too much decision making from him, and perhaps we still do.

Surely it is possible to forge a system that allows for more flexibility in individual rehabilitation, especially if it can be demonstrated that such changes could save money and serve the injured person's needs well. The necessity for a delicate balance in planning rehabilitation services has never been greater. But this discussion of what can be done after injury forgets a most important point, "an ounce of prevention is worth a pound of cure."

Much, much more can be done to prevent brain injury. Children and adults must receive imaginative education about the vulnerability of the brain, the fact that underneath the seemingly impenetrable skull lies this most delicate of organs that controls so much of our total being. There is evidence that education of the public about helmet and seatbelt use and the increasing availability of airbag-equipped cars is lowering the number of brain injuries caused by accidents, but the number of brain injuries caused by gunshot wounds and other violence is up. We read the shocking headlines of children killing children, especially in our cities, but hear very little of those who survive.

LOOKING AHEAD

Like the past, the future holds promise and peril. Will Brian be able to realize his dream of being a nationally known speaker for prevention of brain injuries? Will he be able to become self-supporting, a taxpayer instead of a consumer of disability payments and expensive services? Will he be able to locate (or create) a supported living arrangement and eventually be able to manage his own life? Will he marry, and be capable of parenting? A May 1993 article in Reader's Digest tells the story of a former member of our N. Virginia Head Injury Association support group, Tim Hewitt, who was severely injured in 1981. Tim has been able to sustain a career with the FBI and was married in 1992, accomplishments that must have seemed impossible to his family (and to him) at many points in his long recovery process.

Even when we focus on such positive possibilities, our concerns are many. Our worries are probably similar to those of the families of people with all types of disabilities–physical, sensory, or mental. What will happen to him (or her) when we are gone? What will be the quality of his relationship with his siblings? Will he be able to develop his own support within the community, through friendships, a religious congregation, or helping agencies? What are our responsibilities in providing security for him? What are the variables in a community's ability to know and care about him? Is it money? Is it attitude? Is it the type of community? Do we need to begin now to search out a community with a more clearly demonstrated ability to integrate people with disabilities into the mainstream, through jobs, housing and transportation? A breakthrough on these community issues would certainly ease our minds as we enter our senior years.

I sometimes feel as though we move in a never-ending cycle. Some days we are more accepting of Brian as he is, sometimes we fight the daily realities. When he has forgotten something, we chastise him anew, "Why didn't you write it down?" as if forgetting and not keeping a calendar were surprising new issues! Sometimes we can be in a "letting go" mode, and other times, when he seems to be slipping into isolation or depression, we feel as though we must continue to help him problem-solve.

The community support picture appears fragmented and inefficient at this point. Before Brian moved to Mount Vernon Hospital, many people were working on different parts of him, but no one seemed to see the "whole Brian," until Dr. Gisolfi became his doctor. Similarly, in the present, a host of agencies are meeting various needs, but no one (or group) seems to see the big picture, the cameo of Brian's unique life, and be able to imagine with him ways to move forward. Obstacles to our "letting go" are the inefficiencies and gaps in the present support system here in Northern Virginia, and in Brian's ability to correctly identify the supports he needs.

The bureaucratic solutions to down-the-line challenges of supported living, a decent job, transportation, a social life seldom work well or cost-effectively, in our experience. The local organization that provides services to people with head injury paid for many months $40 a day taxi fare for Brian to get to a job that pays him $40 every two weeks! The problem with this picture–Fastran, the Fairfax County transportation system for people with disabilities, would pick him up for work at the sheltered workshop if he lived in Fairfax County, but could not cross the line into neighboring Arlington County, a territorial ruling that no one has examined for common sense. I could list many more examples. The most effective arrangements are those that are closest to ordinary human experience.

The lasting and caring solutions can only come from the community, and will be increasingly found when people with disabilities *expect* to live an integrated life, whether they live with their families, independently, in group homes, or in nursing homes. Ginny Thornburgh, Director of Religion and Disability of the National Organization on Disability (NOD) believes part of the answer lies in encouraging religious congregations to search their hearts (and their geographical area), looking at ways they can be more welcoming and aware of people with disabilities. There are approximately 43 million Americans with disabilities. Each is primarily *a person* with unique abilities and strengths, and secondarily a person with disability.

Suppose a congregation came to know Brian, and invited him to attend some of their activities–social events for young adults, worship or community service. They would soon discover his unique gifts–his sense of humor, his prevention message to teenagers.

In addition, some very ordinary ways of solving his transportation problems might evolve–a carpool with a commuting member of the church, neighbors who could take turns offering him a ride to the Weekenders social events.

And consider the spiritual benefit to Brian of being warmly welcomed in a caring congregation. Losing the full function of one's mind or body through accident or illness is obviously a painful experience. Sadly, losing friends, losing jobs, losing contact with the world in general is often an unnecessary adjunct to becoming disabled. To make matters worse, some outdated religious attitudes can add to the problem. Imagine being permanently disabled and having a church member say to you, "If your faith had been stronger, you would have been healed long ago." Or hearing someone say as you rolled by on your wheelchair, "There but for the grace of God go I," implying that you are outside the grace of God because you are a paraplegic!

Mary Jane Owen (who is multiply gifted and disabled) of the National Catholic Office for Persons with Disabilities teaches that disabilities are "the normal outcome of the risks, strains and stresses of the living process" and that "pity must be replaced by respectful compassion and mutual recognition of our shared fragility." She encourages us to think of ourselves as "temporarily able-bodied," moving away from the "us and them" framework to greater unity as the people of God.

One creative model of community integration for people with disabilities is called "Circles of Support." Such a circle is a group of people who agree to meet on a regular basis to help the person with a disability accomplish certain personal visions or goals. The focus person may be unable to reach their goals working alone, so asks a number of people–friends, family members, co-workers, neighbors, church members–to form a "Circle." Paid service providers can be an essential resource to the Circle members, but the majority of the members are non-paid, typical community members. One place where Circles of Support are happening is Hartford, Connecticut. Communitas, Inc. has been the guiding light for Circles in Connecticut. According to Pat Beeman of Communitas, there are approximately 100 Circles meeting around the state. Some of these are personally nurtured by Communitas staff and others have sprung up autonomously.

Communitas published an article by Cathy Ludlum, who has been assisted to interdependent living through her Circle. Cathy had wondered if a nursing home would be her only option, when her mother could no longer help with her personal care, "Since respiratory problems are a side-effect of my disability, I have issues around being left alone for anything over an hour." She writes, "I wanted to live where I could feel free and safe at the same time, but could find no such place." Through the support of her Circle, Cathy was able to move into a housing cooperative in 1989 and has the supports she needs for a full life.

I do not intend to imply that this kind of community action can take the place of human services organized by local or national government, but communities must strive for a healthy balance, always with the disabled person's hopes and dreams at the center of any process. Human services organizations are also making a transition to a concept close to that of Circles of Support, calling it "person-centered planning."

● ● ●

I can remember vividly the support of friends over the years, the moments when I was the center of a circle, being guided, helped and carried along through painful events. At other times I sought solitude and silence to draw from deeper wells of the spirit, to be centered on truths beyond my one small life. Later the support of friends often had a different purpose, moving me towards healthy balance, guiding me away from obsession with Brian. Those were the times when my friends needed me to listen with care to the stories of anguish and joy in their lives, getting out of my own small circle. Sometimes the circle is wider still. In The Washington Post in June of 1993, I was startled to see the images of a mother and son in a hospital room overflowing with people wounded in the fighting in Central Bosnia. The 17-year-old boy, dark hair and eyebrows, lay motionless on the pillow, a nasogastric tube protruding from his nostril. By his bedside sat his mother, fatigue and anxiety in her eyes, resting her chin on folded hands. I knew this woman as intimately as if I held her hand.

For my husband and Brian's brothers and sister, I believe there are layers of unexpressed thoughts and feelings–of love, of pain, of adjustment, of anger. Perhaps they will have more opportunities to tell their stories in the future. For now, the moments to be cherished and lifted up are those occasions when we are a family, in the fullest sense. At Scott and Amy's garden wedding in April of 1993, Brian stood by his brother as best man, with Sheri, Eric and Dan also members of the wedding party. Elegant in his tuxedo, Brian seemed thrilled to reach into his pocket for the wedding ring and hand it to Scott at just the right time. At the reception, in his best "public speaker" mode, Brian offered the toast, remembering Scott's enjoyment of Star Trek and the Star Wars trilogy, "Amy and Scott, may the force be with you!"

May the force be with all of us–indeed.

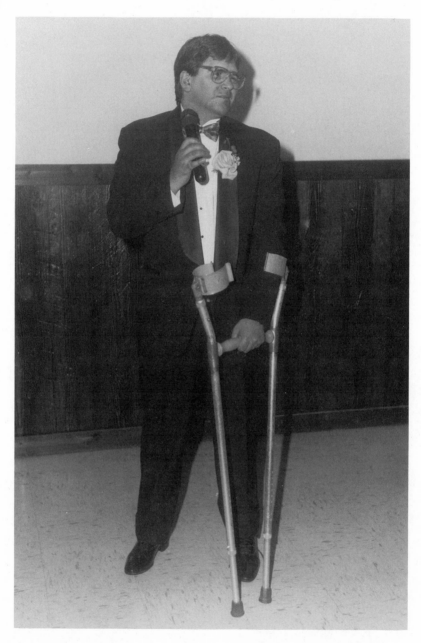

Brian "May the force be with all of us–indeed."

References & Resources

Dufford, B. (1975). Be not afraid. In Limb, No. 497.

Elliott, L. (1988, June). Stand by me. The Washingtonian, p. 131.

Evans, F. (Ed.) (1980). St. Joseph people's prayer book. New York: Catholic Book Publishing Co.

Hagen, C., Malkmus, D., & Durham, P. (1972). Rancho Los Amigos scale. (rev. 1977, Malkmus, D. & Stenderup, K.). Downey, CA: Communication Disorders Service, Rancho Los Amigos Hospital.

Henry, N. (1986, June 8, 9, 10, & 11). Patient No. 18,874. The Washington Post, p. A1+.

John XXIII. (1963). Pacem in Terris. In E. P. DeBerri, P. J. Henriot, & M. J. Schultheis, Catholic social teaching: Our best kept secret (p. 41). Maryknoll, NY: Orbis Books.

Joncas, M. (1979). On eagle's wings. In Limb, No. 448.

Landry, C. (1977). Lay your hands. In Glory & praise.

Levey, B. (1990, May 24). The things that dreams are made of. The Washington Post, p. D10.

Limb, J. J. (Ed.) (1993). Breaking bread 1993: An edition of today's missal. Portland OR: Oregon Catholic Press.

Mazie, D. (1991, June). Keep your teenage driver alive. Reader's Digest, pp. 85 - 90.

Seals, D. (1985). Plant your fields. On K. Lehning. (Producer). Won't be blue anymore. [Audio cassette].

RESOURCES & ORGANIZATIONS

General Disability Groups

Centers for Independent Living (CILs)

CIL's are local organizations, administered and staffed by people with disabilities, that provide peer counseling, advocacy, and information about local services. Call Pat Fairchild, ECNV (703) 525-3462 for number of CIL in your community.

National Information Center for Children and Youth with Disabilities
(NICHCY)
Post Office Box 1492
Washington, DC 20013
(202) 416-0300

National Organization on Disability, (N.O.D.)

910 16th Street, N.W. Suite 600
Washington, DC 20006
(202) 293-596
(202) 293-5968 (TDD)

Well Spouse Foundation

A support group for spouses of people with disabilities.

(914) 357-8513

Brain Injury Support Groups

National Head Injury Foundation (NHIF)

1176 Massachusetts Avenue, NW
Suite 100
Washington, DC 20036
(202) 296-6443 (800) 444-NHIF

Call for phone numbers of state organizations and local chapters. NHIF has a catalog of materials helpful to families and survivors of brain injury. NHIF also publishes a directory of rehabilitatation facilities around the county (because listing is purchased, not all local options are included). NHIF advocates for expanded research, legislative action, and coalition building with other disability groups. NHIF also distributes prevention materials.

<u>Family Survival Project</u>
425 Bush Street
Suite 500
San Francisco, CA 94108
(415) 434-3388

Rehabilitation and Community Re-entry

<u>Accessible Space, Inc.</u>
2550 University Avenue, Suite 301N
St. Paul, Minnesota 55114
(612) 645-7271 (800) 466-7722
A non-profit organization that provides affordable housing and support services for adults with mobility impairments and/or brain injuries.

<u>Independent Living Rehabilitation Program (ILRP)</u>
Al Condeluci, Director of Programs
4638 Centre Avenue
Pittsburgh, PA 15213-1596
(412) 683-7100

<u>Mt. Vernon Hospital Rehabilitation Program</u>
2501 Parker's Lane
Alexandria, VA 2306
(703) 664-7198

<u>Learning Services/Shenandoah</u>
9524 Fairview Avenue
Manassas, VA 22110
(703) 335-9771
Learning Services is a national provider of services for individuals with brain injury, with locations in Georgia, Colorado, North Carolina, Wisconsin, Virginia, California and Utah.

<u>Transitional Learning Community (TLC)</u> at Galveston
P. O. Box 1228
1528 Postoffice
Galveston, TX 775531-800-TLC-GROW

Complimentary videotapes about brain injury: <u>Broken Rhymes,</u> <u>Journey From Flanders,</u> and <u>Mending of the Minds.</u> TLC is one of the best models of brain injury rehabilitation in the country.

Prevention-Oriented Groups

AAA Foundation for Traffic Safety
>1730 M Street, NW, Suite 401
>Washington, DC 20036
>(202) 775-1456

Advocates for Highway and Auto Safety
>777 North Capitol Street, NE
>Suite 410
>Washington, DC 20002
>(202) 408-1711

American Coalition for Traffic Safety
>1110 N. Glebe Road, Suite 1020
>Arlington, VA 22201
>(703) 243-7501

Insurance Institute for Highway Safety
>1005 North Glebe Road
>Arlington, VA 22201
>(703) 247-1500

Mothers Against Drunk Driving (MADD)
>511 E. John Carpenter Freeway
>Suite 700
>Irving, TX 75062
>1-800-GET MADD

National Safe Kids Campaign
>8737 Colesville Road, Suite 100
>Silver Spring, MD 20910
>(202) 884-4993

Spiritual and Community Oriented Groups

Circles of Support: Communitas, Inc.
>P.O. Box 374
>Manchester, CT 06040
>(203) 645-6976

Faith and Light, U.S.A.

Barbara Stevens, Nat'l Coordinator
Rural Route 1, Joshua Cook Lane
Wellfleet, MA, 02667
(508) 349-2514
International association founded by Jean Vanier, of communities of families, friends and persons with mental impairments who meet regularly for prayer, sharing, celebration and pilgrimage. Persons with other disabilities are also warmly welcome.

National Catholic Office for Persons with Disabilities

Mary Jane Owen, Executive Director
P. O. Box 29113 (401 Michigan Avenue, NE)
Washington, DC 20017
(202) 529-2933 (v/TDD)

Religion and Disability Program, Ginny Thornburgh, Director, National Organization on Disability (N.O.D.)

Ginny Thornburgh, Director
910 16th. Street, N.W. Suite 600
Washington, DC 20006
(202) 293-5960, (202) 293-5968 (TDD)

Published interfaith handbook. That All May Worship, to assist congregations in welcoming people with disabilities.

RESEARCH SOURCES

National Institute of Neurological Disorders and Stroke (NINDS)

Supports the work of 12 Head Injury Clinical Research Centers around the country. For information, write:

Office of Scientific and Health Reports
Building 31
Room 8A-16
National Institutes of Health
Bethesda, MD 20892

National Institute on Disability & Rehabilitation Research (NIDRR)

Dr. Paul Thomas
U.S. Department of Education
400 Maryland Avenue, SW

Washington, DC 20202-3430
(202) 205-9194

Rehabilitation Resource and Training Center on Severe Traumatic
Brain Injury (RRTC on STBI)

This group provides an extensive list of useful publications.

Medical College of Virginia
Box 434
Richmond, VA 23298-0434
(804) 786-7290 / (804) 786-0956 (TDD)

Traumatic Brain Injury Centers

A national network of comprehensive regional brain injury research centers, administered by the Rehabilitation Services Administration (RSA), a component of the Office of Special Education and Rehabilitation Services (OSERS), U.S. Department of
Education. For information, contac Timothy C. Muzzio, Ph.D.,
(202) 205-8926

PUBLICATIONS

Books

Chesto, K. O. (1990). Risking Hope. Kansas City: Sheed & Ward.
To order, call: (800) 333-7373.

Condeluci, A. (1991). Interdependence: The route to community.
Orlando: Paul M. Deutsch.

Cumberland Hospital for Children and Adolescents. Pediatric head
trauma guide for families. This booklet can be obtained by writing
or phoning the hospital: PO Box 150, New Kent, VA 23124. (800)
368-3472.

Forest, M. & Snow, J. Support circles: Building a vision. Toronto:
Frontier College. A bibliography of sources on circles of support.
Write to the college at 35 Jackes Avenue, Toronto, Ontario M4T
1E2.

Kushner, H. (1981). When bad things happen to good people. New
York: Random House.

Marshall, L. F., Sadler, G. R., & Marshall S. B. Traumatismo craneo encefalico. New York State Head Injury Association. Order by phone: (518) 459-7911.

Restak, R. (1984). The brain. Toronto: Bantam.

Stearns, A. K. (1984). Living Through Personal Crisis. Chicago: Thomas More Press.

Traumatic Brain Injury Model System Research Program (1993). 1993 Brain injury glossary. Houston: The Institute for Rehabilitation and Research (TIRR). Order by phone: (800) 321-7037.

Periodicals

Exceptional Parent

Parenting Your Child with a Disability
120 State Street
Hackensack, NJ 07601
1-800-247-8080

The Journal of Cognitive Rehabilitation

Bimonthly publication available from NeuroScience Publishers
6555 Carrollton Avenue
Indianapolis, IN 46220

TECHNOLOGY

Neuropage system allows an individual to be reminded of appointments or time to take medication. Neuropage can replace a full time attendant if the attendant serves primarily as a reminder of appointments and commitments. Paging is not stigmatizing. Call Galen Eicher at (800) 279-9700.

Index

Dr. Ommaya. *See* neurosurgeons
Dr. Peter Patrick. *See* neuropsychologist
Dr. Roger Gisolfi. *See* physiatrist
Dr. Schlegel. *See* neurosurgeons
Dr. Wires. *See* neuropsychologist

endocrinologist   88
Ethical considerations   35

facial surgery. *See* maxillo-facial surgeon
Fairfax County Department of Recreation   117
Fairfax County Park Authority   106
Fairfax Hospital   23, 24, 30, 31, 33, 34, 36, 39, 42, 43, 45

Gartlan, State Senator   65
Ginny Thornburgh. *See* Religion and Disability National Organization

Head Injury Foundation   9, 43, 83, 99, 113, 151
Head Injury Rehabilitation Facilities. *See also* Woodrow Wilson
   Lewis Bay in Massachusetts   21
   Vallejo   160

ice water test   37, 38
ICU   15, 25, 28
Images of God   57
Independent Living Rehabilitation Program   103
Intensive Care Unit. *See* ICU

James Kenley. *See* State Department of Health in Richmond

Kaiser-Permanente   14, 34, 39, 43, 46, 62, 65, 82, 83, 159, 160

Ladies of the Club   57
Leesburg Memorial Hospital   43
Louis L'Amour   42, 62, 105

• • •

About the Author and Brian

Janet Miller Rife, a native of Pennsylvania, migrated to Washington, DC as a "government girl" in 1959. During her husband's civil service career, they lived in Hawaii, Belgium, and Virginia, raising five children: Scott, Brian, Sheri, Eric and Dan. Since the early 80's Janet has earned undergraduate credits from the Northern Virginia Community College and from Trinity College in Washington, DC, and an associate degree in religious education through the Education for Parish Service (EPS) program. She served as president of the Northern Virginia chapter of the National Head Injury Foundation 1991-92. Janet lives in Springfield, VA with her husband Curt and their sons Brian and Dan. She currently works as a consultant in the Religion and Disability Program of the National Organization on Disability (N.O.D.) in Washington, is a freelance writer, and an editor/proofreader for EEI in Alexandria.

Brian Francis Rife, born in 1965 in Honolulu, Hawaii, began elementary school in SHAPE (Supreme Headquarters Allied Powers Europe), Belgium, and graduated from St. Bernadette's Catholic School and West Springfield High School, where he was on the wrestling team for three years. Brian played Little League baseball from the 3rd through 8th grades and in the Babe Ruth League in high school. He held various part-time and summer jobs at Longwood College in Farmville, Va before his injury in 1985. Brian currently works two afternoons a week at Wakefield Recreation Center in Annadale, VA, delivers his prevention message to students and driving schools as often as possible, and works on bulk mail at Fairfax Opportunities Unlimited.